To La

MW00758274

LOSE WEIGHT
HEALTHILY

To My New Found
Cousin
I Love you!
To your health

LOSE WEIGHT
HEALTHILY

STOP DIETING AND **START** EATING

LOUISE SMITH

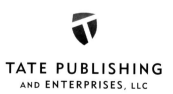

TATE PUBLISHING
AND ENTERPRISES, LLC

This book is designed to provide accurate and authoritative information with regard to the subject matter covered. This information is given with the understanding that neither the author nor Tate Publishing, LLC is engaged in rendering legal, professional advice. Since the details of your situation are fact dependent, you should additionally seek the services of a competent professional.

The opinions expressed by the author are not necessarily those of Tate Publishing, LLC.

Published by Tate Publishing & Enterprises, LLC
127 E. Trade Center Terrace | Mustang, Oklahoma 73064 USA
1.888.361.9473 | www.tatepublishing.com

Tate Publishing is committed to excellence in the publishing industry. The company reflects the philosophy established by the founders, based on Psalm 68:11,
"The Lord gave the word and great was the company of those who published it."

Book design copyright © 2012 by Tate Publishing, LLC. All rights reserved.
Cover design by Shawn Collins
Interior design by Sarah Kirchen
Back cover photo by Jill Jannings—HollandPhoto

Published in the United States of America

ISBN:978-1-61862-301-0
1. Health & Fitness / Diets
2. Health & Fitness / Weight Loss
12.03.12

DEDICATION

This book is dedicated to the Lord of my life, the Lord Jesus Christ.

To LeRoy, my loving husband, friend, and the father of my two beautiful children, who has experienced the ups and downs of life's rollercoaster. Someone who knows and has experienced the power of God's Word and the power of prayer.

To Nathaina, my precious and beloved daughter who is yet a young lady full of wisdom and compassionate. Her love for others has impacted many. I am so proud to be her mother, and I know that God is proud to have her as a daughter.

To LeRoy II, my son who is loving, caring, giving, and who only sees the good in everyone. He has a smile that lights up a room. He is wise far beyond his time. He is the apple of my eye.

To Dr. Gerald K Hill, my friend and brother in Christ, who has always believed in me, whose unfailing support and loyalty has meant a great deal to me.

ACKNOWLEDGEMENTS

I wish to thank my daughter for her patience and understanding and endless hours. This work is a product of her thoughts, ideas, perspectives, and hard work. You are an excellent guide and organizer. You are a writer's dream and a gift to many who will read this work. My accomplishments are your accomplishments. I cherish your life and the part it plays in mine. Thank you for perseverance and always keeping me on track. I love you!

TABLE OF CONTENTS

PREFACE

I strongly believe and hold these facts to be true that my God designed the human body to heal itself. Everything that the human body needs to keep it in perfect health, God provided it on this earth. Absolutely everything man needs is on or in the earth. We do not have to worry about using up the world's resources because the God I know knows the world he created. Do you think that God would create a world without enough? Only man would do such a thing.

It is because of man's disobedience, arrogance, and greed that the people are left wandering around in the "wilderness," searching for something that God has already given, looking for something man made to help us, when, in truth, God has already given it to us.

For decades people have obsessed with the food they eat and, in some cases, the food they do not eat. We are counting calories and not eating the proper foods that have the nutrition that our bodies so badly need. By eating a balanced diet, we will aid our bodies in getting the right nutrients that are required for good health. We have been told for so long that the very foods we need are bad for us. Much has been written concerning the matter of "diet." There are so many sweeping statements, conflicting processes of proof, impossible rules, and foolish conclusions. No wonder you don't know what is good for you. For example, one day, eggs are good, and the next day, they are bad. People take dieting to the extreme and stop eating the very thing that is good for their health and that will control their weight. People are looking for stability in their life and are tired of dieting, being overweight, and not feeling healthy.

All the things you do to lose weight are the very things that make you gain weight. Empty calories, going on strict diets, not getting the proper nutrients are all bad for your health. If you do not get the proper nutrients, you cannot control you weight.

Food is one of the basic requirements for life; without it, you cannot live. It is not only about *what* you eat; it is also about *how* you eat. Food habits are affected by physiological processes, early experiences, ethnic customs, health concerns, social class, and economics. I have linked the Maslow Hierarchy of Needs, the USDA basic food chart, and the Smith's Hierarchy of Nutrition/Nutrients charts to obtain a better understanding.

We must understand certain words in our diet, what they mean, what they do, and what a balanced diet is. In this book I will attempt to explain these concepts to you. I hope you will find yourself in a position to change your life into a healthier lifestyle so that you will have a long quality life.

Well, now you will never have to count calories again. You can maintain your weight and still have a healthy lifestyle. The secret is not what or how much you eat as much as it is about how the body absorbs, digests, or processes what you eat and drink.

Stop dieting, start eating, and lose weight healthy!

INTRODUCTION

This book is a must read for anyone who may have a weight problem or a health problem. It provides the reader with key steps to follow in order to maintain optimal weight and health. Weight has a great impact on health whether it is overweight, obese, underweight, bulimia, anorexia nervosa; no matter which, it all has an effect on health. Body weight can greatly impact your health. Most people know that being overweight (BMI 25-30) or obese (BMI greater than 30) can have adverse effects on your health, but being underweight (BMI lower than 18) also negatively effects your health. Weight management is more than counting calories; it is about energy. It is about good nutrition.

America's health is failing. At an alarming rate, more than half of all Americans have a health problem. Two-thirds of Americans are overweight, and more than 15 million Americans have diabetes. More than 100 million have high cholesterol. To make matters worse, one-third of all America's children are overweight or at risk of becoming overweight. Also, childhood diabetes is growing.

Type 2 diabetes has doubled over the last decade. An estimated 23.6 million people in the United States, roughly about 7 to 8 percent of the population, have diabetes. Of those 23.6 million people, 17.9 million have been diagnosed, and 5.7 million have not yet been diagnosed in 2007. About 1.6 million people ages twenty or older were diagnosed with diabetes. According to the National Diabetes Information Clearing house (NDIC), about 215,000 people younger than twenty years have diabetes type 1 or type 2. This represents 0.26 percent of all people in this age group.

In the United States, as many as 10 million females and 1 million males are fighting a life-and-death battle with an eating disorder, such as anorexia or bulimia. Millions more are struggling with a binge eating disorder. Females between fifteen to twenty-four years old who suffer from anorexia nervosa have a mortality rate associated with the illness that is twenty times higher than the death rate of all other causes of death.

More Americans are becoming overweight or obese, exercising less, and eating unhealthy foods. The latest Gallup-Healthways Well-Being Index shows that 63.1 percent of adults in the US were either overweight or obese in 2009. That was a small but measureable increase from 62.2 percent the previous year. The survey finds that 36.6 percent of Americans are overweight and 26.5 percent are obese.

The Gallup-Healthways Well-Being Index findings are based on telephone interviews with 673,000 adults in January 2008 to December 2009. About 90,000 surveys were done each quarter, and the margin of error for the quarterly results is +/-0.3 percentage points.

The survey finds that:

- 59.2 percent of obese Americans exercised at least one day per week, compared to 69.9 percent of overweight people, and 73.8 percent of normal-weight people.

- Obese people are less likely than people in every other weight category (overweight, normal weight, underweight) to have eaten five servings of fruits and vegetables on at least three days of the past seven.

- Obese Americans also are less likely to say they ate the recommended five servings of fruits and vegetables three to seven days per week:

- 71.6 percent of normal-weight people

- 69 percent of underweight people

- 68.9 percent of overweight people

- 67.2 percent of obese people

Body mass index (BMI) is a common measure of body fat based on height and weight

The survey found that:

- Of people with high blood pressure, 46.2 percent were obese, 31.1 percent were overweight, 19.3 percent were of normal weight, and 17.2 percent underweight.

- Of people with high cholesterol, 36.8 percent were obese, 30.1 overweight, 19.2 percent normal weight and 14.1 percent underweight.

- Of people with diabetes, 21.1 percent were obese, 9.8 percent overweight, 5 percent normal weight, and 4.2 percent underweight.

- Of people reporting heart attacks, 6.3 percent were obese, 4.8 percent overweight, 3.3 percent normal weight and 4.4 percent underweight.

- Of depressed people 23.3 percent were obese, 15.3 percent overweight, 15 percent normal weight, and 20 percent underweight.

The survey says that African-Americans in 2009 were among the most likely to be obese at 36.2 percent, compared to the national average of 26.5 percent. The obesity rate among Hispanics, at 28.3 percent, is also higher than the national average. Asians are far less likely to be obese, with only 9.6 percent falling into that category.

The survey also reports that 18.3 percent of young Americans are obese, compared to 27.6 percent between ages thirty to forty-four and 30.6 percent among forty-five- to sixty-four-year-olds. Of people sixty-five and over, 24.2 percent are obese. Men are more likely than women to be obese—27.8 percent compared to 25.2 percent.

All these issues come down to the *food* or nutrition/nutrients that your body receives. By reading this book, this could help you with the problem up front. After all, sickness and disease comes from what we put into our bodies or what we do not put in our bodies.

I spent three years performing research on health issues. The information presented in this book is a collaboration of studies published by the NIH and from many scientists. While most studies or scientists focused on only one subject, I took the information and combined it in one source. I am a health advocate with years of health experience stemming from my time as a nurse, Army medic, EMT, and president of a community health clinic.

For more information, visit www.rywhe.com.

STOP DIETING, START EATING, AND LOSE WEIGHT

Have you ever seen a skinny person drinking or eating diet food? Well, have you? Probably not. Why? Because it doesn't work! Look at the word diet. What is left after you remove the T…Die! That's right; dieting is slowly killing you.

We should rely upon our food to provide us with important nutrients, as well as be our energy source. Omitting meals and certain foods or food groups can be the beginning of a downward spiral of the physical and mental functions of our body. An inadequate intake of nutrients can cause a reduction in our physiological function, leading to poor health.

To constantly be in dieting mode is a dysfunctional state of mind. You cannot afford to accept anything but the highest standard of physiological and biological excellence as normal. Anything short of this structure, and the highest vigor and efficiency of function must be recognized as a state of impaired health. You should make food your medicine. To live by medicine is to live horribly, for it is not living at all; it is merely existing and being in a dysfunctional state.

Life is a tragedy of nutrition; the lack of the proper nutrition is the cause of all diseases and imperfect health of any kind. Elimination of foods to lose weight is not good. For starters, dieting does not work; it is only temporary, and if you do it frequently and for long periods at a time, it can cause serious damage to your physical health as well as to your mental health.

All diseases of the body are due to the lack of certain food principles, such as mineral salts, vitamins, or the absence of the normal defenses of the body, like the natural protective flora, enzymes, and probiotics. When this occurs, toxic bacteria invade the lower alimentary canal, and the poisons thus generated pollute the bloodstream and gradually deteriorate and destroy every tissue, gland, and organ of the body.

Promise yourself that you will never again go on a diet. They do not work. You always feel like you are missing something, you are not eating the nutrients that you need, and they never last. So come on. Say out loud, "I will never go on another diet, and I will lose and have a stable weight." You did not say it; this is what your have been looking for all of your life.

What is Nutrition?

Nutrition is the science that links foods to health and disease. It includes the processes by which the human organism ingests, digests, absorbs, transports, and excretes food substance.

Nutrients

Nutrients are chemical substances in food that contribute to health and are essential parts of a diet. Nutrients nourish us by providing calories to fulfill energy needs, materials for building body parts, and factors to regulate necessary chemical processes in the body.

Nutrients come from food.

What is the difference between food and nutrients? Food provides energy in the form of calories, as well as the materials needed to build and maintain all the body cells. Nutrients are the substances obtained from food that are vital for growth and maintenance of a healthy body throughout life. For a substance to be considered an essential nutrient, three characteristics are needed. It must be a vital organic dietary substance that is not an energy-producing carbohydrate, fat, or protein. It is usually necessary in only small quantities to perform a particular metabolic function or to prevent an associated deficiency disease. Lastly, it cannot be manufactured by the body and therefore must be supplied in food.

There are six food groups:

1. Carbohydrates

2. Lipids (fats and oils)

3. Proteins

4. Vitamins

5. Minerals

6. Water

It is important to know that no one nutrient works alone; however, they work in concert, synergistically, with other nutrients. One may set the stage for the activity of another or work in unison with them, while some neutralize or balance the effects of others. Each nutrient is discussed individually and more in depth in subsequent chapters.

Dieting is not healthy because you are taking a risk of not getting the nutrients that you need for your body, the body needs nutrients to function properly, and dieting does not allow for your body to receive the proper nutrients that it needs. People who diet a lot are shortening their days because dieting ages them, as well as causes sickness and disease. Nutrients come from the food you eat and drink, so therefore, when you go on long diets, you deprive yourself of the proper nutrients that you need. No one can stay on a diet all of their lives unless they want a short life. Therefore, we need to learn how to stop dieting and start eating healthy and balanced meals in order to maintain a healthy weight for our bodies.

Eat Your Way to Perfect Health

Eat your way to perfect weight and health by eating food. This is no gimmick or a game being played; it is true. Eating right is vital to promoting health and reducing the risk for death or disability due to chronic diseases such as heart disease, certain cancers, diabetes, stroke, and osteoporosis. In fact, according to the government's dietary guidelines for Americas 2005, it has been estimated that by eating balanced meals, we could reduce cancer deaths in the United States by as much as 35 percent.

By the way it is not how many calories you are eating, so stop counting calories and start counting nutrients. Okay, I know that you can't count nutrients exactly; however, you can take notice of the nutrients that are in the food that you are eating. I know you say, "How am I supposed to do that?" I am glad that you asked! If what you want to eat is natural and raw, like a vegetable, a fruit, and/or a whole grain, then it is full of nutrients. There is no need to count calories; just know that nutrients are there.

Weight maintenance is all about energy balance and good nutrition. It isn't about elimination of foods from your diet or about not even eating snacks but rather about balancing the composition. The number one thing to remember is to have a balanced diet. All of our energy comes from the food we eat and what we drink, mainly carbohydrates, fats, and proteins. Your meals should provide your body with all of the basic nutrients that it needs to provide you with energy each day as well as to repair and build tissue.

Your meals must consist of a combination of protein, (good) fat, carbohydrates, along with anything else that you are eating. This will allow your food to work for you and not against you. Having your food work for you means that your foods are working together to ʾuce energy and burn fats. At every meal, in mod- ˑ, you must have—number one—some type of protein. Second, a good form of carbohydrate. Lastly, eat some (good) fat, along with fiber and whatever else you may eat. Make this a combination even with your snacks. The big "no" in your diet is having *fructose* in your food, even if you eat refined foods, please eat in moderation and eat more fiber. Fiber will slow down the simple carbohydrates and turn them into energy instead of fat storage. Fats are not the reason that you are overweight; fat burns fats.

Stop counting calories and focusing on what and how much you are eating. Start focusing on the nutrients in the food that you are eating; it is not about the number of calories as much as it is about what the body is doing with it once you eat. What is essential is how the body reacts to the food you eat. Does it digest or absorb it? Is it slow or fast? Does it use it for energy or does it store it as fat? How your body processes what you eat is so important. Knowing what the right combination of foods to eat at each meal and even at snack time is essential to stability in weight and in good health.

If what science and the USDA say is true, potatoes are not bad for you; as a matter of fact, they are very good for you. I have read many articles that say that potatoes are bad for you; this is not so. How can something that has as many nutrients as potatoes do be bad for you? I think that this is said because they are white. It is how you prepare the potatoes. Do you deep-fry them in oil full of trans fats? What is the portion size? What toppings are you using? Your answers are probably what is bad, not the actual potato. Below are the vitamins and minerals found in one medium potato, according to the Department of Agriculture Food and Nutrient Center:

MINERALS		VITAMINS	
Potassium	962mg	Vitamin C	16.6mg
Phosphorous	121mg	Niacin	2.439 mg
Magnesium	48mg	Vitamin B1	0.111mg
Calcium	26mg	Vitamin B2	0.083mg
Iron	1.87mg	Pantothenic Acid	0.65mg
Sodium	17mg	Vitamin B6	0.538mg
Zinc	0.62mg	Folate	48mcg
Copper	0.204mg	Vitamin A	0.17iu
Manganese	0.379mg	Vitamin K	3.5mcg
Selenium	0.7mcg	Vitamin E	0.07mg

Also contains other minerals and vitamin in small amounts.

Energy Balance

Energy balance is the difference between the calorie intake from food and drinks and the metabolic energy expended during daily activity. In order to lose fat/weight, our body needs to be in a negative energy balance. Negative energy balance must be a consistent, gradual process. There will always be natural changes in physiology in order to constantly balance energy within the body. Changes are driven by what we eat, when we eat, and how much we eat. The source of energy available to the body comes from solid food plus fluids (such as milk and juice).

Dieters count calories, but the amount of weight loss doesn't add up. Weight loss confusion occurs because there is a physiological adaptation to under eating in order to balance energy within the body and help maintain weight quickly. Every time we eat, a certain amount of energy is used to digest and absorb all the nutrients. Most diets naturally require a reduction in food intake, so less food eaten means less energy is required to maintain weight. This process is known as the "thermic" effect of food.

Eating less also means fewer nutrients available for maintenance of muscle tissue, especially protein needed for synthesis of antibodies or enzymes. These are molecules that are in constant need twenty-four hours a day, and a constant supply of protein must be maintained. If no protein is consumed, then there is a gradual loss of protein from muscle cells in order to maintain a healthy immune system. A net protein loss naturally reduces lean weight, which lowers the metabolism. The end result is lowered energy expenditure, rendering the present, low-calorie diet ineffective.

There are several ways in which the body expends energy; one is the basal metabolic rate (BMR). The BMR is the total amount of energy expended when the body is apparently at rest. BMR refers to the work of breathing, contraction of the heart, circulation of the blood, kidney function, the metabolism of all the body's living cells and in the process of digestion, and absorption of foodstuffs.

After a meal, the processes of digestion and absorption are initiated and continue for some hours.

Negative calorie foods are foods that use more calories to digest than the calories the food actually contains! So by eating foods that are low in calories yet take longer to digest, the body will actually be using more calories than the food has in order to process the foods. These extra calories required for digestion are taken from fat stores in the body. The more of these negative calorie foods that are eaten, the more weight will be lost.

Calories from these foods are much harder for the body to use. In other words, the body has to work hard in order to extract calories from these foods. Even though a food may contain an equal amount of calories, much fewer of these calories can possibly turn into fat in negative calorie foods, as fewer calories are actually available to the body; this gives these foods a tremendous, natural, fat-burning advantage. See negative/fating burning food list.

BALANCED DIET

It's Not the Food

From a nutritional standpoint, the beauty of taking whole, natural food is that it provides a full spectrum of nutrients, and you can be certain that your health is being optimally supported. Vegetables, fruits, whole grains, and beans are low in calories, and full of fiber, vitamins, and minerals. These foods may reduce your risk of cancer, heart disease, and kidney disease and help you to lose weight. Whole and natural organic foods are full of health-promoting potential that is nutrient rich. We should rely upon our food to provide us with important nutrients. It is important to know that nutrients do not work alone but in conjunction (synergistically) with other nutrients. It is important not to focus on a single nutrient intake but on intake of an array of nutrients.

It is not the food that you are eating that is making you fat or gain weight; it is the additives that are in the food. Additives such as high fructose corn syrup (HFCS) and refined white sugar are in all refined, processed food. Make sure that there is no high fructose corn syrup in your diet. I know that it is hard to do since just about everything has fructose added. Please avoid HFCS, and if you must eat it, flush it with fiber. Fruit has natural fiber. Fiber slows the absorption of sugar. There is something about fructose, sugar, and diet foods and drinks that make you always feel hungry, never satisfied, always wanting more. You remain thirsty, and therefore, you are always drinking and consuming empty calories.

When making choices about the right kind of foods to eat, we normally make the wrong choice based upon misinformation about what we should or should not eat. Leaving out food groups can lead to an incomplete diet and slowly lead to sickness and disease as well as premature aging. Most diets are incomplete. Incomplete diets cause weight gain and health problems because taking very important nutrients out of your diet is not good.

Balanced Diet

Is your body using food for energy, or is it storing food for fat? If your food is balanced, the body will use it for energy every time. Eating a balanced diet is about what the body does with the food you take in; make your food work for you and not against you. To have food working for you is when you turn carbohydrates, fats, and protein into energy. The combination will speed up your metabolism by making the digestive system work hard, creating a fat-burning machine. Having a balanced diet is to have stability or have equilibrium.

The importance of a balanced diet throughout life cannot be underestimated. Instead of saying that we are what we eat, maybe we should say that we are what we absorb. According to Dr. Edward Howell, the prevention of chronic and life-threatening illness, rapid recovery from sugar or disease, and optimal physical and psychosocial functions depend on the ingestion of necessary amounts of carbohydrates proteins, fats, vitamins, minerals, and fluids.

Your body requires protein, carbohydrates, and fats, and it needs them in large amounts to perform basic cellular functions. These are called macronutrients. When planning your meals, always make sure that you have a balanced diet. This means that you provide your body with all of the basic nutrients that it needs to provide you with energy each day. A balanced diet must contain carbohydrate, protein, fat vitamins, mineral salts, and fiber. It must also contain these things in the correct proportions.

If you are always feeling tired and feeling like you need to have something to pick you up just to get you going then you need to check your diet. Ask yourself if you are getting the right amount of the right kinds of energy source foods. According to the NIH, you need to get between 45 to 65 percent of your energy should come from carbohydrates, and 35 percent should come from fats—the good fat, which I will show you later.

A balanced diet should consist of fruits, vegetables, whole grains, legumes, fats carbohydrates, and proteins. When eating your meals or favorite foods, make sure that you eat them in moderation and in a combination of carbohydrates, protein, and fats. Also eat a food high in fiber, such as an apple. The fiber, fat, and protein will slow the absorption of the fruit sugars into the blood stream. For most people, especially those with diabetes and insulin resistance, this is a good thing. Fiber and protein in particular reduces the glycemic effect of high glycemic fruits such as bananas and strawberries.

Example: For a meal you should eat a combination of foods, like a sandwich of lean meat, whole wheat bread, a piece of fruit, and some raw vegetable of choice. For a snack you should eat peanut butter crackers or cheese crackers with an apple or another piece of fruit or celery.

Plate:

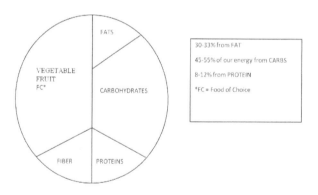

On the plate there are carbohydrates, proteins, fats, fiber, and natural sweets. Also see list on fast-burning foods as well as a chart on a list of combination foods to choose from.

When you eat a meal with of a combination of fats, protein, carbohydrates, vitamins, mineral salts, and fiber all in moderation, you will be less likely to gain weight. Eating a meal that omits carbohydrates or proteins will make you more likely to gain weight and not feel well. The body needs a mixture of a balanced diet to aid with absorption. The way the body absorbs the nutrients determines our well being. For calcium to absorb, you need a combination of other minerals and vitamins, such as phosphorus, magnesium, manganese, fat, and vitamin D. If you are missing one of either one of these, you will not have the full affect of calcium; therefore, it could have an effect on your bones, teeth, heart, and nerves. They all work together; they do not work alone. They need each other.

You Are What You Eat

This is a true saying; you are what you eat. It is impossible to live without food; the reason that we cannot live without food is that all of our natural vitamins, minerals, and energy come from the food we eat. Vitamins and minerals are vital for life. Despite their importance, however, the human body is not equipped to produce all the vitamins and minerals it needs to function. Instead, these nutrients must be obtained from food. Vitamins and minerals must be absorbed by the body before they can be used effectively.

Don't remove the essential nutrients out of your diet and think that will be better for you. The key nutrients are carbohydrates, proteins, and fats because they are important for the proper function of our bodies.

Do not skip meals. Do not diet. Eat in moderation. Stay away from diet foods. Diet foods have a tendency to create cravings by making you hungry, and you never feel full; therefore, you will eat more of the wrong foods, which will be converted to fat. This is unhealthy. You will eat lot of empty calories.

When making a choice, you should try to stick to foods that are *raw, natural, whole bran,* and *no preservatives* as much as possible. Stay away from items that are refined, white, processed, and synthetic. If you follow these examples, you will not only lose weight; you will maintain your weight, and you will also notice that you will tone. So it is not about not eating; it is about eating and eating yourself to a slimmer and healthy vigorous you.

CALORIES

A calorie is a unit of measurement for energy. Calories are in anything containing energy, not just foods. In scientific terms, a calorie is the amount of energy or heat it takes to raise the temperature of one gram of water by one degree. A calorie measures the energy amount in the food and beverages you consume.

Everything we do relies on the energy that comes in the form of calories. Our bodies need that energy to live. Some calorie consumption is essential, a must, and vital for life processes. Human beings need energy to survive, to breath, to move, and to pump blood, and we acquire this energy from the food we eat. Carbohydrates, protein, and fats all contain calories, while vitamins and minerals, including antioxidants and fiber, do not contain calories.

Empty Calories

Empty-calorie foods are foods that are very high in calories but low in nutrients. This is food with high calorie content and no nutrients and leads to weight gain and poor health. This food type does not have any substance that can assist the body in its proper function. Empty calorie foods usually have high levels of high fructose corn syrup and white sugar and are highly processed foods.

"Junk foods" are a classic example of empty foods. These are any foods with little enzyme production, no vitamins, and no mineral content. The ingestion of empty calorie foods requires the body to use its own enzymes (usually found in the lining of the intestinal tract) to be able to convert these empty calories into usable energy. Obviously, these enzyme-producing functions in the body should be reserved for the performance of other internal and more vital metabolic reactions.

This is just the reason that dieting doesn't work, because most people eat food with no nutrients. It is true that you may lose weight; however, you will not get the nutrients your body needs, and you will lose weight in an unhealthy way.

NEGATIVE CALORIE/ FAT-BURNING FOODS

It is hard work for the body to breakdown food; absorb all the protein, carbohydrates, fats, vitamins, and minerals; and then release the unused portion from the body. Certain types of foods require a lot of energy/calories to breakdown, be absorbed, and be used inside of the body. Some of these foods contain very few overall calories and, therefore, may actually force the body to call upon the energy stores in the form of stored glucose and fat to finish processing the food.

There are several ways in which the body expends energy, most importantly:

1. The basal metabolic rate (BMR)

2. The processes of digestion and absorption of foodstuffs (Yes, eating burns calories)

3. Physical activity

The BMR is the total amount of energy expended when the body is apparently at rest. BMR refers to the work of breathing, heart contractions, blood circulation, kidney function, and even includes the metabolism of all the body's living cells. If the average woman did nothing except stay in bed all day, she would still burn between 1,200 to 1,400 calories a day. For the average man, he would burn around 1,700 calories per day.

After a meal is consumed, the processes of digestion and absorption are initiated and continue for some hours. So that being said, by eating the right food, you can actually lose weight and be in perfect health. Physical activity obviously affects energy expenditure. However, you could lose more weight by eating the right food and the right combination of foods. For example, if you eat a piece of pie with 300 calories, you would have to run three miles to burn it off. And for every pound you lose, you would have to burn 3,500 calories. Three thousand five hundred calories is the rough estimate for the energy contained in one pound of fat. This means in order to lose one pound per week, you must create a deficit of 3,500 calories per week. This equals about 500 calories per day.

Negative *value* foods or empty-calorie foods are foods that are full of empty calories with no nutrients. Negative calorie foods are foods that use more energy/calories to digest than the amount of calories present in the foods. All foods have some calorie content. No food actually has negative calories. It is the overall effect of digesting certain foods in our body that makes it have negative calories.

Calories from what we call negative-calorie foods are much harder for the body to breakdown and process. In other words, the body has to work harder in order to extract calories from these foods. This gives these foods a tremendous, natural, fat-burning advantage. It is known that our bodies use up energy in digesting food. In fact, it is believed that about 10 percent of calories from a meal are burned up while your body digests and processes the foods.

Dietary fiber, also known as roughage, includes all parts of the plant that the body cannot digest or absorb. The crunchier and the bulkier the roughage, the more energy it takes to digest it. Using this theory, if you eat one hundred calories of vegetables that require 150 calories to digest, then you've burnt an additional fifty calories simply by eating that food. Whereas a piece of dessert consisting of 400 calories may use 150 calories for digestion but results in a net gain of 250 calories, which is added to our body fat!

Fiber is classified in two categories: soluble fiber and insoluble fiber. Soluble fiber dissolves in water to form a gel like material. As a result, your body receives the nutrients of enzymes, probiotics, vitamins, and minerals. These nutrients do not have calorie content. Insoluble fiber is the fiber undigested by your digestive system and promotes movement of material through the digestive system as well. The insoluble waste of fiber passes relatively intact, through your stomach, small intestine, colon, and out of the body, flushing with it fats and toxins. This is why fiber is great for weight loss and great health.

So it stands to reason that you can eat all of the green vegetables you want and still lose weight. Nevertheless, you must remember to have a balanced diet. A balanced diet is essential. Along with all of those vegetables, make sure you have small portions of protein, fat, and carbohydrates; you need energy along with nutrients in order to lose and maintain your weight and be in good health. The ingestion of empty-calorie foods requires the body to produce its own enzymes (usually in the lining of the intestinal tract) to be able to convert these "empty calories" into usable energy. Obviously, these enzyme-producing functions in the body should be reserved for the performance of other internal and more vital metabolic reactions.

Surprisingly, in the case of the negative-calorie foods, they not only contain sufficient vitamins and minerals to break down the host calories, there is actually a surplus of these enzyme-producing biochemicals. This simply means that once ingested, these negative-calorie foods provide for enzyme production in quantities sufficient to break down not only its own host calories but possibly additional calories present in the digestive tract as well.

Vegetable Negative Calorie List:

- Asparagus

- Fennel

- Aubergine

- Broccoli

- Leek

- Cabbage

- Lettuce

- Carrots

- Marrow

- Cauliflower

- Peppers

- Celery

- Radish

- Chicory

- Spinach

- Cress

- Tomato

- Cumber

- Turnip

- Beet

- Chile peppers (hot)

- Cucumber

- Endive

- Dandelion

- Garlic

- Green beans

- Onion

- Radish

- Garden cress

- Greens

- Kale

- Red cabbage

- Green vegetable or fibrous vegetable

Fruit Negative Calorie List:

- Apricot

- Mandarin orange

- Apple

- Cranberries

- Grapefruit

- Lemon

- Raspberry

- Plums

- Pineapple

- Tangerine

- Mango

- Melon

- Cantaloupe

- Peaches

- Orange

- Guava

- Strawberry

Natural starch, carbohydrates or whole grain, brown rice, oats, and sweet potatoes have a very strong effect on the metabolism. Also dry beans, of all kinds.

Most lean meats help to speed up the metabolism and burn more fat, simply because they require so much energy for digestion. Omega-3 fats, the healthiest of good fats, also alter levels of a body hormone called leptin. Cold-water fish and omega-3 oils are definitely strong fat-burning food substances.

Meat:

- Chicken breast

- Lean beef

- Turkey

- Pork

- Lamb (lamb has an amino acid (icarnitine), which is natural in the body and has impact on fat)

Fish:

- Salmon

- Tuna

- Sardines

- Shrimp

- Cod

- Scallops

- Herring

- Cold-water fish

- Farm-raised fish

*Salmon, tuna, sardines, and herring contain large amounts of omega-3 fatty acids as well as have a strong effect on metabolism.

TIPS TO MAINTAIN WEIGHT LOSS

1. Eat all the foods you like; however, do so in moderation. Make sure the bread and pasta is whole grain.

2. Make sure that the food you eat has no preservatives or anything that is not natural.

3. No fructose or sucrose at all. You will begin to lose weight quickly just by removing these unnatural sugars from your diet.

4. If you must have something sweet, and it is not fruit, then look for evaporated cane juice, organic raw sugar, or molasses. These types of sugars do not go through heavy processing and still contain nutrients and are natural.

5. Eat food in combination at every meal, and eat in moderation.

Basic:

First eat a piece of fruit like pineapple, papaya, or mango. These fruit choices have enzymes that help start the digestive system.

Meat about the size of a deck of cards

Vegetables

A whole-wheat carbohydrate, as this will push fats and waste through the digestive tract and be less likely stored as fat.

Lunch example:

- Pineapple

- Macaroni and cheese

- Chicken breast

- Green vegetables

- Slice of whole wheat bread

Dinner example:

- Mango

- Spaghetti and meat sauce or meat balls

- Garlic bread

- Vegetable of choice

Or:

- Papaya

- Tuna steak

- Brown Rice or whole grain pasta

- Greens of any kind

- Dessert in moderation

If you must have something sweet, make sure you eat something with a large amount of fiber. This will slow the sugar and not let it become fat storage. With this kind of meal, you will have a slow carbohydrate and a fast carbohydrate, fat, and protein. This combination enables the food to work for you and not against you.

See list on combination of foods to combine for loss of weight. Also, you must be more active. Exercise does not have to be excessive. You can just park your car farther away from the exit or take the stairs instead of the escalator. Walk more and add additional steps. If you cannot afford to go the gym, clean your own house, as this increases the amount of movement you will do throughout the day. More exercise is very important, not just for the fact it will help you lose weight, but more so that it helps keep you in good shape.

Beauty is but the reflection of wholeness, of health" (Dr. Herbert Shelton, 1968).

Love Yourself

Stop just existing and begin to live life. Life is short, and you only get one. Stop spending your time doing the things that take away from your life like starting diets again and again, all the while inadvertently harming yourself. Having illness, disease, depression with eating disorders, whether it be excess eating, anorexia, bulimia, or binge-eating affects our well being.

Remember, love yourself and appreciate the body that God has given you. Embrace yourself; feel good about the space that you are in. If you love it, others will too. Beauty is how you feel about yourself. And by the way, real women have curves. Your weight should be according to the (USDA) height/weight guidelines. I believe that if you are ten to fifteen pounds overweight, it is not so bad; or if you are ten to fifteen pounds under, it is not so bad. However, if your weight goes outside this ten-to-fifteen-pound weight range in any direction, it can be detrimental to your health. To be too much overweight or underweight can be serious; after this point, your health is in jeopardy, and you must immediately try to change it.

Use this height and weight chart as a guideline. It is also important to make your perfect weight according to your body frame.

HEIGHT/WEIGHT GUIDELINES

WOMEN				MEN		
	low	midpoint	high		low	midpoint
4'10"	100	115	131	5'1"	123	134
4'11"	101	117	134	5'2"	125	137
5'0"	103	120	137	5'3"	127	139
5'1"	105	122	140	5'4"	129	142
5'2"	108	125	144	5'5"	131	145
5'3"	111	128	148	5'6"	133	148
5'4"	114	133	152	5'7"	135	151
5'5"	117	136	156	5'8"	137	154
5'6"	120	140	160	5'9"	139	157
5'7"	123	143	164	5'10"	141	160
5'8"	126	146	167	5'11"	144	164
5'9"	129	150	170	6'0"	147	167
5'10	132	153	173	6'1"	150	171
5'11	135	156	176	6'2"	153	175
6'0'	138	159	179	6'3"	157	179

English measurements: Height is in feet and inches and weight is in pounds

Your meals should be balanced with vitamins, minerals, fats, proteins, carbohydrates, and fiber. If you eat food that contains these things, you will be able to control your weight. Go ahead, eat! Do not skip meals, as this causes your metabolism to slow down; you must eat. However, you must remember the word *moderation*.

DANGER OF FRUCTOSE AND HIGH FRUCTOSE CORN SYRUP (HFCS)

Sugar is a term usually used to refer to table sugar or sucrose. Sugar can also be used to refer to crystalline carbohydrates of varying sweetness, including glucose, fructose, and lactose just to name a few.

Refined white sugar, the table sugar that most people use every day, is harmful, even in small amounts. Refined sugar is an extremely high-glycemic food. It hits your bloodstream hard and can have severe impact on blood sugar levels, insulin levels, digestive enzyme count, weight, and the pancreas. Anything that has been chemically changed, refined, processed, or has color changes are manufactured and are not good for you. Refined white sugar is unhealthy. Consuming refined sugar is one of the worst things you can do to your immune system. White sugar suppresses the immune system. According to Natural Medicine, white sugar has been shown to decrease the vitality and number of white blood cells, the body's immune response to invaders. Sugar also depresses the body's energy field and makes your blood more acidic, both of which result in vulnerability to toxins, bacteria, and viruses. Sugar feeds bacteria, like Candida, which causes yeast infections. Anything that says it is sugar, sweetener, and has been changed is not natural, and the body does not process it. Therefore, it will do harm to the body, causing sickness and disease.

However, not all sugars are unhealthy. Certain sugars have minimal or no negative impact on the body and actually have remarkable health benefits. Evaporated pure cane juice still has most of its nutrients such as minerals. Evaporated cane juice does not undergo the same modification process as refined white sugar. Organic whole sugar is also unrefined, unbleached, whole cane sugar that is sun dried and evaporated into pure, golden-brown crystals.

Natural sugar in fruit, called fructose, is a good sugar as long as it is in its *natural* state. Fructose from fruit is found in *fresh fruit* only. Natural fructose is not made into a sugar-like substance in the body; do not get them mixed up. The fructose found in the ingredients of your processed food is *not* the same fructose that stems from fresh fruit. If fructose is in your food as an additive, it is not from fruit and, therefore, not natural.

Dr. Robert Lustig, MD, a pediatric endocrinologist and professor at the University of California, San Francisco, states that the fructose that comes in nature, like from a piece of fruit or sugar cane, is consumed along with its fiber.[1]

Fiber slows down the absorption of sugar, and fruit has so many other nutrients. The fiber plays a critical role in suppressing our insulin response and in causing our satiety signal to kick in sooner, so we don't eat as much.

In actuality, your body needs *natural* sugars in order to stabilize the system. Don't listen to the hype that fruit sugars are not good for you. Fruit is one of the healthiest things you can eat. Natural fruit juice can be one of the best things you can drink as long as it is fresh and has nothing added.

Fructose

Unnatural fructose is directly metabolized by the body into abnormal fat. A high "fat" diet is actually filled with unnatural fructose, as stated by Dr. Lustig. Please note that when I refer to fructose from this point, I mean the unnatural fructose and not the natural fructose from fresh fruit. Fructose is a high fat diet.

That fact that fructose drives fat storage and makes the brain think that is hungry is a vicious cycle and is what makes fructose so harmful. Fructose is a component of the two most popular sweeteners: table sugar and high fructose corn syrup (HFCS). There is no difference between table sugar and high fructose corn syrup, as both are a combination of glucose and fructose—meaning, when the body metabolizes table sugar (sucrose) and HFCS, they are broken down into fructose and glucose. Fructose is a toxin that only the liver can process. Glucose, the standard sugar, can be taken up by every organ in the body. Only 20 percent of glucose ends up at your liver (Lustig).

Fructose and glucose are *not* the same. Glucose is the energy of life, as it is needed in almost all bodily processes; fructose is a slow death. The only organ that can take up fructose is your liver. Fructose has the same effect on the liver as alcohol does. Dr. Lustig claims that fructose is just as bad as alcohol because it causes fat storage in the liver and can cause fatty liver disease. He also states that fructose is like alcohol but without the buzz (Lustig).

Dr. Lustig states, "Fructose is a poison." Fructose consumption changes the way your brain recognizes energy. Unfortunately it is all in a negative fashion. Essentially, fructose makes you think that you are starving. Your brain gets the signal that you are starving even though your fat cells are all generating signals that you are full. Fructose suppresses ghrelin, the hunger hormone. As a result, we tend to eat more. Also fructose has been shown to interfere with the leptin signal, which causes you to eat more. Fructose has a chronic effect, not an acute effect. This chronic effect has to do with years of fructose-saturated meals or a lifetime's worth of fructose meals. Eventually you become insulin resistant.

Ghrelin is a hormone that controls appetite, increases the secretion of growth hormones, and even affects the function of the brain. It appears to play a large part in neurotrophy, which is the influence of nerves on nutrition and maintenance of body tissue. In addition, ghrelin is important in helping the brain make cognitive adaptations and other changes in response to environment. Therefore, it is critical to the learning process.

Could this be in part having something to do with our children with learning disability, attention deficient, autism, and even Alzheimer's in our older people? It is possible that this has something to do with the high rate of all of these illnesses in our society.

Leptin is a hormone that is tied closely to regulating energy intake and expenditure, including appetite, metabolism, and hunger. It is the single most important hormone when it comes to understanding why we feel hungry or full. When present in high levels, it signals to our brain that we're full and can stop eating. When low, we feel hungry and crave food. It does this by stimulating receptors in our hypothalamus, the part of our brains that regulates the hormone system in our bodies. When leptin binds to receptors in this part of our brains, it stimulates the release of appetite-suppressing chemicals. People with leptin disorders eat uncontrollably.

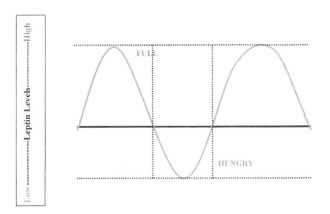

The above chart shows that, at low leptin levels, your brain thinks that you are hungry. This leads to increased eating habits.

The bad news is that excess weight can lead to leptin resistance. Shapiro et al 2008 published a study in the American Journal of Physiology found that high fructose diets can induce leptin resistance (National Institutes of Health State-of-the-Science Panel). These sugars actually impair leptin's ability to cross the blood-brain barrier and reach the hypothalamus. This means that even when the leptin levels are high, not enough leptin is reaching the brain in order to tell the body to stop eating. As a result, you end up looking like the person on the right:

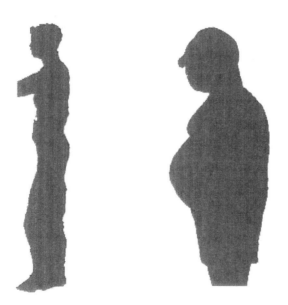

The person on the right is the result of impaired Leptin signals.

Lustig's groundbreaking studies more than a decade ago stimulated the development of his controversial ideas about metabolism and biological feedback in weight control. One not-yet-popular idea is that calorie-for-calorie sugar causes more insulin resistance in the liver than other edibles. The pancreas then has to release more insulin to satisfy the liver's needs. High insulin levels, in turn, interfere with the brain's receipt of signals from leptin, secreted by fat cells.

Eating stimulates secretion of insulin and leptin. Insulin, like leptin, has a feedback system to the brain that limits food intake. Elevated insulin levels block leptin's negative feedback signal. Lustig believes that fructose generates insulin resistance more than other foodstuffs. Therefore, fructose calories fail to blunt appetite in the same way as other foods. As a result, the body tends to grow more obese.

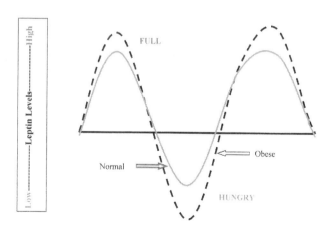

Fig. shows how a change in leptin levels can make you obese.

Chronic fructose exposure is associated with eight of the same health outcomes as chronic alcohol exposure. Drinking a can of soda is like drinking a can of beer. They are both linked with hypertension, myocardial infraction, dyslipidema, pancreatitis, obesity, hepatic dysfunction (Nonalcoholic steatohepatitis NASH), fetal insulin resistance, and habituation /addiction.

Fructose metabolism creates fatty acids, which assemble as fat droplets in the liver and muscles tissue. These fat deposits lead to a non-alcoholic, fatty liver and insulin resistance, which, in turn, can progress to metabolic syndrome. Metabolic syndrome is a combination of two or more of the following diseases: obesity, type 2 diabetes, lipid problems, hypertension, and cardiovascular disease. A waste product of fructose metabolism is uric acid, which has been shown to increase the risk of grout and hypertension.

High Fructose Corn Syrup

Table sugar is 50/50 fructose and glucose. High fructose corn syrup has varying percentages of fructose ranging from 42 percent to 90 percent. For example, HFCS-55 is 55 percent fructose and 45 percent glucose and is used in most soft drinks (Lustig). You know, the commercials are right; there really is no difference between sucrose (table sugar) and high fructose corn syrup. High fructose corn syrup and sucrose are virtually the exact same; they are both equally bad and they are both like poison in high doses.

High fructose corn syrup is not from fruit. No matter what people say, it is not from fruit. So what is high fructose corn syrup? HFCS is a man-made sweetener that is found in a wide range of processed foods, from ketchup and cereals to crackers and salad dressings. The HFCS used in foods is usually between 50 to 55 percent fructose—so chemically, it's virtually identical to table sugar (sucrose), which is 50 percent fructose.

High fructose is an extremely highly over processed substance, and it is put into highly processed foods—a double whammy. This cannot be good for you, as it has absolutely no value. High fructose corn syrup destroys your liver and causes weight gain, obesity, diabetes, hypertension, and atherosclerosis.

High fructose corn syrup came on the market after it was invented in Japan in 1966 and started finding its way into American foods in 1975. In 1980, soft drink companies started introducing HFCS into drinks. You can actually trace the prevalence and rise of childhood obesity to 1980 when the change to HFCS was made. Dr. Lustig states, "This so alarming and frightening, our consumption of fructose has gone from less than half (1/2) a pound per year in 1970 to 56 pounds per year in 2003" (Lustig). The solution to losing weight or to preventing obesity is to keep this poison out of our food. There is no drug that can cure obesity. However, there is a chemical that can cause obesity, and it is high fructose corn syrup.

Barry Popkin, PhD, a Nutrition professor at the University of North Carolina at Chapel Hill, suggested in an influential 2004 paper, a possible HFCS-obesity link. This paper stresses that the real obesity problem doesn't lie just with HFCS. Rather it's the fact that sugars from all sources have become so prevalent in our food supply, especially in our beverages. He scoffs at the "natural" sweeteners sometimes added to upscale processed foods like organic crackers and salad dressings. "They all have the same caloric effects as sugar," he explains. "I don't care whether something contains brown sugar, honey, or HFCS. The only better sweetener option is none of the above."

According to Dr. Edward Group's website, Global Healing Center natural health, and Organic Living there are five health dangers of high fructose corn syrup (Group);

1. Significant risk of weight gain and obesity:

The list of studies that show HFCS to cause increased weight gain over other forms of sweeteners is much too long to put into this post. A recent study conducted at Princeton University found that rats that were fed HFCS gained fat 300 percent more quickly than those fed an equal (or slightly larger) dose of fruit-derived sugar.

2. Increase risk of developing type 2 diabetes:

Over the years, consumption of high fructose corn syrup can lead to a huge increase in the likelihood of developing diabetes. The worst part about it is how easily this lifelong condition can be avoided in most cases.

3. Hypertension and elevated bad cholesterol levels

High fructose doesn't just make your body fat; it makes your heart fat too. There is a strong link between the irresponsible consumption of high fructose corn syrup and elevated triglyceride and HDL (bad cholesterol) levels. Together these can cause arterial plaque buildup. Eventually this leads to dangerous heart conditions, including hypertension, heart disease, and even stroke.

4. High fructose corn syrup and long-term liver damage

Liver damage from HFCS consumption is a major danger that a lot of people overlook. Like anything else you eat or drink, HFCS is processed by your liver, gallbladder, and kidneys. It is especially destructive to your liver. When combined with a sedentary lifestyle, permanent liver scarring can occur. This greatly diminishes the organ's ability to process out toxins. Over time this can lead to an expansive range of other negative health concerns. Another study suggests that HFCS may also cause fatty liver.

5. Mercury exposure from HFCS

Even if you were already aware of previously mentioned risks associated with corn syrup, there's a good chance that you didn't know it is also often loaded with alarmingly high levels of mercury. In a study conducted in 2009, they found mercury in over 50 percent of the samples tested. Mercury exposure can result in irreversible brain and nervous system damage, especially in young, growing bodies. This is especially worrisome with the abundance of HFCS in children-targeted foodstuffs.

I know you will be hard pressed to find food that does not have HFCS, but you must try to limit yourself to as little as possible. You should go into grocery stores and ask them to get food that is absent of these additives.

I personally believe that HFCS is habit forming. It is no different than having an addiction to crack cocaine. Adults are like babies, always having a bottle in their mouths. People feel as though we cannot do without sweets. You just have to have the sugar fix, whether it is in a soda or something sweet to eat. In the end, you feel like you have not eaten. You crave for something sweet. That is why HFCS is put in everything, even foods that should not be sweet, such as chips. Think about it; why can't you have just one, as one chip brand used to advertise?

No matter what the food is, if it contains high fructose corn syrup, it is unhealthy even when you think you are eating healthy options, such as yogurt. I know right now you are panicky, thinking, *How can I not eat sweets?* This thought is just another sign that you have become addicted to it. Have no fear; I will give you a list of sweeteners that you can use but that you still must use in moderation.

High fructose corn syrup and sucrose (table sugar) are equally destructive; they both contain fructose, which can only be metabolized by the liver, poisoning it and making it insulin resistant. This insulin resistance in the liver can cause chronically raised insulin, which makes us feel badly and store fat. HFCS stimulates our appetite and interferes with leptin signals to the brain, so we eat more.

There is nothing natural about fructose; don't let the name fool you. HFCS is manufactured using genetically modified organisms (GMOs). It is not natural. It is a man-made ingredient. Avoid HFCS at all costs. In fact, HFCS leads to all the manifestations of metabolic syndrome, including inflammation, hypertension, bad cholesterol, obesity, fatty liver, and leptin resistance. Note that these consequences do not take into account GMO corn used in HFCS or that mercury is found in HFCS.

In nature, fructose is always found with lots of fiber and other essential nutrients. However, high fructose corn syrup is not found in nature and is added to almost all processed foods, which already have all nutrients removed.

SLOW-BURNING VS. FAST-BURNING FOODS

Slow-burning foods are foods that stay in the stomach longer, thereby making you feel fuller longer. This cuts down on cravings, and it takes more energy to digest. When it takes more energy to digest, it also burns calories. These foods help burn calories without any extra workout time. Fast-burning foods are foods that provide us with immediate energy. They quickly enter the blood and cause a sharp insulin spike. Although fast-burning foods provide us with energy, they do not burn calories and are more likely to be stored as fat.

Carbohydrates are the most important and ready source of energy in our body. Forty-five percent to 65 percent of our energy should come from *complex carbohydrates* because they are digested more slowly than simple carbohydrates and are less likely to be converted to fat. Complex carbohydrates must be part of your daily diet for a balanced diet.

Always include in your meals a fast carbohydrate, slow carbohydrate, and a healthy fat. This combination ensures that the synergy among them helps the body to turn carbohydrate, proteins, and fats to energy rather that to store it as fat. The combination forces the digestive system to work harder, which means that it is producing energy rather than just storing it as fat. The harder the digestive system works to break down food, the better it is for you because it is producing energy, burning fat, and *not* storing fat.

Slow-Burning Foods:

- Eye of round

- Lean ground beef

- Sirloin

- Tenderloin

- Top loin

- Top round

Poultry:

- Turkey bacon

- Turkey breast

- Chicken breast

- Baked chicken

- Chicken fried in olive oil

Pork:

- Broiled ham

- Canadian bacon

- Loin

- Tenderloin

Legumes:

- Beans

- Italian beans wax

- Black-eyed peas

- Black bean

- Broad beans

- Butter beans

- Cannelloni beans

- Chickpeas or garbanzo

- Kidney beans

- Great northern beans

- Lentils

- Lima beans

- Pigeon

- Soy beans

- Split peas

- White beans

- Pinto beans

Seafood:

- All Types
- Eggs (use egg white and/or the whole egg)

Oils:

- Olive oil
- Coconut Oil
- Flaxseed oil
- Sunflower seed oil

Vegetables:

- Artichokes
- Asparagus
- Broccoli
- Bok choy
- Cabbage (red and white)
- Cauliflower celery
- Collard greens
- Cucumbers
- Eggplant
- Lettuce (all varieties)
- Tomatoes

- V-8 juice

- Mushrooms

- Mustard greens

- Okra

- Red onion

- Peppers (all varieties)

- Pickles, dill

- Radishes

- Rhubarb

- Sauerkraut

- Snow peas

- Spinach sprouts

- Alfalfa

- Squash (various types)

- Zucchini

Soy Substitute:

- Bacon, burger, chicken, hot dogs, sausage links or patties, tofu

Seasonings:

- (Any that contains *no* added sugar)

- Broth

- Espresso

- Power extracts (vanilla, almond, etc.)

- Horseradish sauce

- Butter

- Smart balance spray

- Lemon juice

- Lime juice

- Mustard

- Pepper (black, cayenne red, etc.),

- Salsa

- Hot sauce

- Steak sauce

- Worcestershire sauce

Nuts (just a few for snacks):

- *Eat dry roasted

- Almonds

- Brazil nuts

- Peanuts

- Cashews

- Pecans

- Macadamia

- Peanut butter

- Almond butter

- Pine nuts

- Pistachios

- Walnuts

Dairy:

- Low-fat milk

- Fat-free milk

- Soy milk

- Almond milk

- Half and half

Treats:

- Fudgesicles

- Gelatin

- Popsicles

Fast-Burning Foods:

- Green peas

- Jelly and jams of (all varieties)

Grains:

- Millet

- Steamed white rice

- New potatoes

- White bread

- Pastry (all varieties)

- Boiled rice

- Brown rice

Dairy:

- Ice cream

- Yogurt

- Skim milk

- Whole milk

Fruit:

- Basically all fruits because they have a natural sugar

- Watermelon

- Pineapple

- Raisins

- Mango

- Oranges

- Pears

- Peaches

- Grapefruits

- Grapes

- All varieties of fruit juice*

- *If you are not careful, you can and probably drink most of your calories without evening thinking. This can cause weight gain. Absorbing empty calories adds unhealthy sugar to our diet, which can be a big problem.

Junk Food:

- Chips

- Candies

- Sugary drinks, such as soda (all sugary drinks)

*Basically anything that dissolves quickly into the blood stream.

Remember at every meal/snack, combine a fast carbohydrate, a slow carbohydrate, and a healthy fat along with your meal in moderation. This is what I call negative foods/fat-burning food, and you will not only see weight loss but toning as well.

Create Your Plate

Vegetables [1]

Spinach
Swiss chard
Asparagus
Broccoli
Collard Greens
Kale
Mustard green
Brussels sprouts
Green Beans
Summer Squash
Bell peppers
Cauliflower
Green peas
Cabbage
Carrots
Beets
Beet Greens [2]
Sweet potatoes
White potatoes
Corn
Avocados
Spinach with Scalloped Onions [2]
Caulifower [3]

Grains

Oats
Granola with fruit and nuts
Oat meal
Rye
Rye stuffed cabbage
Rye wrap
Quinoa cereal with fruit
Quinoa wrap
Grits
Brown rice
Sesame rice
Rice pudding
Sea vegetable rice
Vegetable sushi rolls
Wheat
Whole wheat with berries
Buckwheat
Buckwheat tabouli
Cornbread [5]
All Noodles [6]

Fruit /Deserts

Strawberries
Strawberries and mints
Strawberries parfait
Strawberries with cashew sauce
Strawberries with orange sauce
Strawberries with chocolate crème
Raspberries
Raspberries almond parfait
Raspberries with balsamic vinegar
Raspberries with lemon sauce
Raspberries with yogurt and chocolate
Cantaloupe
Cantaloupe with lime and mint
Cantaloupe sorbet
Cantaloupe fruit salad
Cantaloupe melon balls
Pineapple
Pineapple fruit salad
Pineapple shish-ka-bobs
Pineapple shrimp salad
Pineapple chicken salad
Kiwifruit
Kiwi with lemon sauce
Oranges
Oranges and avocado salad
Orange salsa
Orange granite
Orange French toast
Papaya
Papaya with lime
Papaya fruit cup
Papaya chicken salad
Ginger papaya salad
Green papaya salad
Papaya smoothie
Watermelon
Watermelon kiwi soup
Watermelon jicama
Watermelon granite
Apricots
Apricots fruit cup
Apricot bar
Grapefruit
Grapefruit salad
Grapefruit sunrise
Grapefruit arugula salad
Grapefruit salsa
Grapefruit granita
Grapes
Grapes with yogurt salad

Fish and shellfish

Tuna
Broiled Tuna steaks
Classic shrimp Scampi
Salmon quick broiled salmon
Salmon with ginger mint salsa
Miso salmon
Salmon with dill sauce
Egg salmon salad
Steam salmon
Salmon frittata
Cod
Quick broil
Mediterranean cod
Cod tacos
Sweet and spice cod
Cod with herbs
Sardines
Sardines with Dijon caper sauce
Sardines with papaya
Sardines with garlic
Sardines on salad fresh broiled sardines
Scallops
Healthy sautéed scallops
Mediterranean scallops
Scallops poached in orange juice
Poultry and lean meats
Calf's liver
Calf's liver and onions
Liver spread
Grass feed beef
Venison sautéed with peppers
Lamb chops
Rosemary quick broiled lamb
Lamb with Dijon mustard
Lamb burger with yogurt
Roasted turkey
Romaine turkey wrap
Tortilla free wrap
Turkey hash
Turkey with ravigote Sauce
Chicken baked
Broiled chicken
Curry chicken
Olive oil fried chicken

Beans and Legumes

Lentils
Lentil soup with curry
Vegetables soup with lentils
Pureed lentils
Soy beans
Whole soy bean pod
Kidney beans
Kidney beans romaine wrap
Kidney bean pasta
Kidney bean taco
Cajun kidney beans chili
Pinto beans
Pinto bean chili
Pureed pinto beans with poached egg
Chili Pasta
Lima beans
Mediterranean Lima beans
Mexican succotash
Lima bean soup
Pureed lima beans
Black beans
Black bean breakfast wrap
Black bean soup
Black bean chili
Black bean and butter squash
Black bean burrito
Garbanzo beans
Mediterranean Garbanzo Beans
Hummus wrap
Garbanzo bean soup
Miso tofu soup
Mediterranean   tofu
Sweet firecracker tofu
Sweet and sour tofu
Split peas
Asian flavor peas
Split pea with kale and spinach
Navy beans
Pureed navy beans
Italian navy beans soup
Navy bean pesto dip

Curried Waldorf salad
Grapes with honey-lemon sauce
Raisins
Raisins fruit compote
Raisins butter
Raisins trail mix
Blueberries
Blueberries with yogurt
Blueberry – peach yogurt
Blueberry with cashew-almond sauce
Cranberries
Cranberry and fresh pear cobbler [4]
Oatmeal with cranberries
Green salad with cranberries
Cranberry spritzer
Cranberry trail mix
Prunes
Prunes and almond treat
Spiced prunes with yogurt
Prunes with lemon sauce
Apples
Apple –carrot salad
Baked apples
Figs
Figs stuffed figs with cheese
Figs and almond treat
Fresh pears
Pears with ginger topping
Pear and water cress salad
Pears and millet porridge
Pears with lemon sauce
Pears with almond –cashew crème

Salads

Rainbow salad [7]
Caesar   salad
Toss salad
Tuna Salad
Chicken salad
Egg salad
Avocado salad
Peanut shrimp salad
Shrimp salad
Tuna salad
Pinto bean corn salad
Garbanzo bean salad
Rye spinach salad
Soba noodle salad
Quinoa salad
Spinach salad
Green salad

Sandwich [11]

Tuna
Tuna salad
Chicken
Chicken salad
Egg salad
Cucumber and tomato
Cucumber and tomato salad
Sardines [10]

Oils and herbs and spices

Oliver oil
Coconut oil
Flaxseed oil
Avocados oil
Omega -3, omega-6 oil [9]
Parsley
Mustard seeds
Basil
Turmeric
Cinnamon
Cayenne/red chili peppers
Black pepper
Ginger
Dill
Cilantro
Rosemary

Snacks [8]

Nuts and seeds
Sunflowers seed
Flaxseeds
Pumpkin seeds
Walnuts
Almond
Peanut
Cashews
Pecan
Papaya seeds
Walnuts
Sesame seeds

Milk and cheese
Almond milk
Soy milk
Goat's milk
Goat cheese
Feta cheese
Butter milk
Plain yogurt [13]

Soup
Creamy carrot soup [12]
Tomato Soup
Beet Soup
Sweet Potato Soup
Split Pea Soup
Black Bean Soup
Vegetable Soup

1. Remember when preparing only sauteé lightly and watch the dressing that you used on foods find a more healthy way to give food a good taste. Do not use unhealthy fats or sweetness that can cause harm. Preparation is a big process.

2. Sauté

3. Sauté with Olive oil and Lemon juice

4. With organic evaporated cane juice sugar (no white sugar or refined sugar)

5. Natural Cornmeal

6. Whole Wheat

7. red cabbage, white cabbage, carrots, celery, beets, red onions , white onions, radish, peppers: red, green, orange, yellow

8. remember all nuts and seeds must be dry roasted and no additives

9. from Fish like Salmon, Sardines

10. Chopped with papaya

11. On Whole Wheat Bread

12. Use Almond Milk

13. Only using fresh fruits and nuts

FATS

Fat does not make you fat; fat burns fat, converting it into energy.

Fats are organic compounds that are made up of carbon, hydrogen, and oxygen. They are a source of energy in foods. Fats belong to a group of substances called lipids that come in a liquid or a solid form. The function of fat is to supply calories or energy to the body along with protein and carbohydrates. Fat is essential for the proper functioning of the body. They are important for bodily functions, such as controlling inflammation, blood clotting, and brain development. Fats fill cells, which make adipose tissues that help insulate the body.

Functions of Fat

Fats provide energy. Gram for gram, fat is the most efficient source of food energy.

Fats build healthy cells. Fats are a vital part of the membrane that surrounds each cell of the body. Without a healthy cell membrane, the rest of the cell cannot function.

Fats build the brain. The brain is 70 percent fat. Fat provides the structural components not only of cell membranes in the brain but also of myelin, the fatty insulating sheath that surrounds each nerve fiber, enabling it to carry messages faster.

Fats make hormones. If what science says about this is true, then women need more fat to assist with the menstruation cycle as well as to assist them with menopause when they get older. I also believe that it may also help sexual libido stimulation for women and men. Fats are structural components of some of the most important substance in the body, including prostaglandins, hormone-like substances that regulate many of the body's functions. Fats regulate the production of sex hormones, which explain why some teenage girls who are too lean experience delayed pubertal development and amenorrhea.

Fats maintain healthy skin. Healthy skin and hair are maintained by fat. Fat helps the body absorb and transport the vitamins A, D, E, and K. One of the more obvious signs of fatty acid deficiency is dry, flaky skin. In addition to giving skin its rounded appeal, the layer of fat just beneath the skin (called substances fat) acts as the body's own insulation to help regulate body temperature. Lean people tend to be sensitive to cold; obese people tend to be more sensitive to warm weather.

Fats protect your organs. Fats form a protective cushion for your organs. Many of the vital organs, especially the kidneys, heart, and intestines, are cushioned by fat that helps protect them from injury and hold them in place. True, some of us "overprotect" our bodies. As a tribute to the body's own protective wisdom, this protective fat is the last to be used up when the body's energy reserves are being tapped into.

There are *three* kinds of fats in the human body.

1. Structural Fat: It surrounds the organs and joints. It is important for protecting the organs and arteries and keeping the skin smooth and taught. It also provides cushioning under the bones of the feet and joints.

2. Normal Fat: It is the normal fat reserves used as fuel when the body is dealing with nutritional or calorie insufficiencies. This is spread all over the body. Structural and normal fat reserves are in fact normal and needed for good health. Interestingly enough, when people do any type of diet and exercise weight reducing regimes, it is this fat plus muscle that is lost. This is why people who lose weight with every other diet and exercise program have a sore heel, sore feet, sore joints, develop arthritis, and have sagging, old-looking skin. They are losing important structural fat, some normal fat, and important muscle mass.

3. Abnormal Fat: It is abnormal, secure reserves of fat. This third fat is a reserve of fuel, but unlike the normal, readily accessible fat reserves spread throughout the body, this fat is located in what is called the "problem areas." In women this is most often

the hips, thighs, and buttocks. In men it is most often the waist and upper chest. This fat is stored as a survival mechanism and is only released in the most severe nutritional emergency when the body is close to near starvation. It is also released during pregnancy to ensure the survival of the unborn fetus. In obese patients, the body abnormally stores most of its fat reserves in these areas. This creates a grotesque disfiguration of the body shape and guarantees that the person will virtually find it impossible to lose weight in the future.

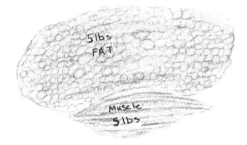

Fat takes up more space than muscle.

*Fat vs. Muscle Diagram

The words *oil, fat,* and *lipids* are used to refer to different forms of fats. *Oil* is the word used in reference to fats that are liquids at room temperature. *Fat* is the word used to reference fats that are a solid at room temperature. *Lipids* is used to refer to both liquid and solid fats, along with other related substances.

All fats are combinations of saturated and unsaturated fatty acids. External fats provide essential fatty acids, which are not made by the body and must be obtained from food. The essential fatty acids are linolenic acid and alpha-linolenic acid. Most importantly to brain function are the two essential fatty acids, also called omega-6 (linolenic) and omega-3 (alpha-linolenic). These fatty acids are the prime structural components of brain cell membranes to transport valuable nutrients in and out of the cells.

Smart Fats

Fats make up 70 percent of the brain and nerves that run every system in the body. So it stands to reason that the more fat in the diet, the better the brain. So with all the fat eaten by the average American, why don't we have more geniuses in this country? The American brain is getting fat, but it's not getting the right kind of fat.

The body needs two types of fat to manufacture healthy brain cells: the message senders, and prostaglandins, the messengers. One type is omega-6 fatty acids, which is found in many oils, such as safflower, sunflower, corn, and sesame oils. The other is omega-3 fatty acids found in flax, pumpkin seeds, walnuts, and cold-water fish, such as salmon and tuna. The foods from which oil can be extracted are generally the foods highest in essential fatty acids.

When the cells of the human body and the human brain are deprived of essential fatty acids, they need to grow and function, the cells will try to build replacement fatty acids that are similar but may actually be harmful. Higher blood levels of "replacement fatty acids" are associated with diets that are high in hydrogenated fats and diets that contain excessive elevated in persons from depression or attention deficit disorder. A diet rich in omega-3 fatty acids, such as the LNA from flax oil or EPA and DHA from fish oils, not only provide the body with healthy fats but also lowers the blood level of potentially harmful ones, such as cholesterol and possibly even reversing the effects of excess trans acids.

With that said, it is so important to have the *right kind* of fat in your diet. Studies have shown that most Americans eat a lot of the wrong kind of fat. It is essential that you know what the right fats are and eliminate all the wrong fats from your diet. Remember that fat does not make you fat; fat burns fat.

Types Of Fat

Good

Monounsaturated fats—fats found in oils and plants—have been shown to decrease total cholesterol and LDL cholesterol and maintain HDL cholesterol. Monounsaturated fat always comes in a liquid from. It is very good for your health because it lowers the bad and increases the good cholesterol. The most popular source of monounsaturated fat is olive oil. When deciding what kind of baking fat to use, you should go for olive oil and leave the other baking fat on the shelves.

Sources:

- Olive oil

- Flaxseed oil

- Arachis oil (peanut oil)

- Cashew nuts

- Peanuts

- Almonds

- Avocado

- Coconut

Polyunstaturated Fats—fat found in oils, nuts, fish, and plants. Polyunsaturated fat contains the essential fats, omega-3 and omega-6. It lowers our bad cholesterol and raises our good cholesterol, just like monounsaturated fat. Omega fats should play a very important part in your diet, as your body cannot make these by itself.

Omega-6: Polyunsaturated fats have been shown to decrease risk for heart disease by decreasing total cholesterol and LDL cholesterol.

Omega-6 fat sources:

- Safflower oil

- Grape seed oil

- Sunflower oil

- Walnut oil

Omega-3: Fats from fish have been shown to reduce the risk of cardiac arrhythmia and sudden death. The modes of action are not fully understood but are due in large part to anti-inflammatory/antithrombotic capacity.

Omega-3 fat sources:

- Flaxseed oil

- Walnut oil

- Soybean oil

- Fish oils

- Fatty fish oils

It is important to know that your omega-3 and omega-6 fat intake must be well balanced.

Bad

Saturated fat—fat found in animal food and processed foods, which utilize oils that are high in saturated fat. Studies show that too much saturated fat in person's diet increases heart disease risk by increasing total cholesterol and LDL cholesterol.

Trans fat—fat formed during the process of hydrogenation, which helps to keep oils solid and stable at room temperature for use in foods. It is also found naturally occurring in small amounts in meat and milk. Increases heart disease risk but is thought to be even more harmful because not only does it increase cholesterol, but it decreases HDL cholesterol as well.

Coconut oil has been given a bad name! Coconut oil is a saturated oil. However, it is not even in the same class of other saturated oils; it is in a class of its own. Coconut oil is considered saturated only in name because it comes in a solid form. Because coconut oil has natural content and the fact that it is from a plant, which has many benefits, it is one the oils that should be used. There are very few, if any, oils that have as many nutrients as coconut oil. If you look at the nutrients in coconut oil, you will see that coconut oil is actually good for you. Look at the nutrients in unrefined coconut oil:

- Fiber

- B-vitamins

- Vitamin C

- Iron

- Potassium

- Phosphorus

- Protein

- Fat

- Carbohydrates

How can something with this many nutrients have anything that would harm you? Dr. Bruce Fife, a Naturopathic Medial Practitioner, calls coconut oil the healthiest oil on earth (Group). Coconut oil represents the richest source of medium chain fatty acids, natural compounds that provide a number of effects in the human body. Dr. Fife explains that these fatty acids, which take their name from the yeasts, bacteria, and viruses. Like Dr. Fife, I believe in the benefits of coconut oil and how good it can be for your health. I personally use it and love it. It also gives food a good taste without increasing additives.

The main component in coconut oil, almost 50 percent, is lauric acid. According to Dr. John J. Kabara, professor Emeritus of Michigan State University, lauric acid is found in nature in such an abundance only in breast milk. Lauric acid is a medium chain fatty acid that is antiviral, antibacterial, and used to destroy lipid-coated viruses such as those found in HIV and herpes, according to the international wellness directory website.

Fat Deficiency

If you don't have enough fat in your diet and body, you can develop:

- dry, scaly skin

- hair loss

- low body weight

- cold intolerance

- bruising

- poor growth

- lower resistance to infection

- poor wound healing

- loss of menstruation

Fat helps the body produce endorphins (natural substances) in the brain that produce pleasurable feelings. Diets too low in fat (less than 25 percent) may trigger cravings. Due to the fact that fat helps food to stay in the stomach longer, giving a greater sense of satisfaction, that prevents hunger soon after meals. This may prevent cravings, which could possibly help with weight loss. Fat does not make you fat; fat burns fat, converting it into energy.

Fat is *not* the problem. The problem is fructose, high fructose corn syrup, and GMOs.

ENZYMES

Dr. Edward Howell, the father of Enzyme Nutrition, says that enzymes are the substances that make life possible (Howell). They are needed for every chemical reaction that occurs in our body. Without enzymes, no activity within the body would take place. Vitamins, minerals, and hormones cannot nourish the body without working in conjunction with enzymes.

Enzymes are energized protein molecules found in all living cells. They catalyze and regulate all biochemical reactions that occur within the human body. They are also instrumental in digestion. They break down proteins, fats, carbohydrates, and fiber, making it possible to benefit from the nutrients found in those foods while removing the toxins. Enzymes turn the food we eat into energy and unlock this energy for use in the body. The presence and strength of enzymes can be determined by improved blood and immune system functions.

No person, plant, or animal can exist without enzymes. They are all run by metabolic enzymes. Enzymes are the manual workers that build our body from proteins, carbohydrates, and fats, just as construction workers build our homes. Enzymes are involved in all bodily functions. Every activity that occurs within the body involves enzymes: the beating of the heart, the building and repairing of tissue, the digestion and absorption of food—it goes on and on. Nothing can occur without energy, and energy cannot be produced or used without enzymes. Without enzymes, there would be no breathing, no digestion, no growth, no blood coagulation, no perception of the senses, and no reproduction. Our bodies contain trillions of enzymes, which continually renew, maintain, and protect us.

Each enzyme promotes one type of chemical reaction and one type only. Some enzymes help break down large nutrient molecules (the proteins, carbohydrates, and fats in our foods) into smaller molecules for digestion. Others are responsible for different functions, such as the storage and release of energy or the processes of respiration, vision, etc. Did you know that enzymes combat the aging process by increasing the blood supply to the skin? Increased circulation helps to bring nutrients to the skin, and it also helps take away the waste products that can make the skin look dull and wrinkled.

It is essential to know that there are three types of enzymes: *metabolic*, *digestive*, and *food enzymes*. Commonly we only think of the digestive enzymes because they make it possible for our body to break down and absorb the food we eat. Our bodies naturally produce metabolic and digestive enzymes as they are needed. Food enzymes can only be consumed orally (by mouth).

Metabolic enzymes speed up chemical reactions occurring within cells for detoxification and energy production. They enable us to see, hear, feel, move, and think. Every organ, every tissue, and all 100 trillion cells in our body depend upon the reaction of metabolic enzymes and their energy factor. Metabolic enzymes are produced by every living cell. However, the liver, pancreas, gallbladder, and other organs play a vital role in their production.

Digestive enzymes are secreted along the digestive tract to break food down into nutrients and waste. This allows nutrients to be absorbed into the blood stream and the waste to be discarded. Human digestive enzymes include ptyalin, pepsin, trypsin, lipase, protease, and amylase. Digestive enzymes play a major role in breaking down food into nutrients that can be absorbed by your body. The body does not make cellulose, an enzyme necessary for proper digestion of fiber, so it must be introduced through the raw foods we eat.

Food enzymes are introduced to the body through the raw foods we eat. Raw foods naturally contain enzymes, providing a source of digestive enzymes when ingested. However, each food enzyme only helps to digest a particular substance. For example, the lactase enzyme can only digest lactose (a milk sugar) and cannot systemically support another substance such as protein. The cooking and processing of food destroys all the enzymes in the food. Each food product contains only enough enzymes to process that particular food, so our bodies must produce the majority of the digestive enzymes we require.

In order to benefit from eating well, your body has to properly digest and absorb the nutrients from your food. The human produces digestive enzymes that break down the food you eat into nutrients. Nutrients are then absorbed into your body through the small intestine. Enzymes are important because they assist in the digestion and absorption of food. They are known to be the life force and/or energy of food.

A human is nourished and maintained not by what he/she eats but by what is digested. All food is at least potentially a poison until converted into simple structures by enzymes. There are two types of life-building chemistries. One type is called exogenous, and it is found in raw food. The other type is referred to as endogenous enzymes, and they are produced within your own body. The more enzymes one gets from exogenous sources like raw food, the less will have to be supplied by the pancreas and leukocytes, thus allowing endogenous enzymes to be utilized for the body maintenance, waste disposal, and extension of longevity.

A diet rich in enzymes can increase energy and stamina as well as support weight loss, healthy skin, and overall good health. Eating complex carbohydrates, fresh fruit, and vegetables (which are loaded with activating enzymes) allows the natural sugars to enter the bloodstream slowly, resulting in a more gradual and longer-lasting buildup of energy.

How can some people eat nutritious foods and yet be continually tired, develop chronic disease, and/or age prematurely? Quite possibly, it could be due to poor digestion and/or poor absorption of foods. In other words, an individual could be eating a healthy diet, but the nutrients aren't getting to the body. Literally one can eat the best diet and yet the body is starving.

Digestion begins in the mouth with your saliva by breaking down the carbohydrates and fats in your food. Good digestion begins in the mouth with the chewing process. The action of chewing starts the production of digestive enzymes in your stomach. Chewing rejuvenates your digestive system. In order for enzymes to do their job, we must chew well. By chewing well, you help the enzymes in the mouth to attack your food. This makes the food more digestible and exposes more of the food surface to enzymatic juices.

The more time you spend chewing, the more surface area of the food will be exposed to enzymes, leading to better digestion. Chewing is especially important for raw vegetables and fruits. Most raw fruits and vegetables have cellulose membranes, which must be broken before nutrients can be released and the food can be digested.

All carbohydrates (sugar, starch, vegetables, and fruits) require an alkaline environment in order to have the best enzymatic reaction. This alkaline environment occurs in the mouth. Carbohydrates need to be thoroughly chewed. Therefore, begin by putting small portions of food or the amount of food you can chew properly in your mouth at a time. Remember, undigested food is like poison. You should never put so much in your mouth that you have to swallow before you chew. Don't put anything else into your mouth until you have completely chewed and swallowed everything already in your mouth.

Enzymes are responsible for breaking up the starches, fat, and proteins that we eat. Once the food molecules have entered the stomach, the stomach enzymes work to break it down further. Proteins, fats, and carbohydrates are broken down in preparation for the absorption. The food is then moved into your small intestines, where most of the absorption process takes place. The lining of the intestines produces more enzymes to break down fats, carbohydrates, and proteins. There are three enzymes found in the small intestine. They are protease, lipase, and amylase. These enzymes help you get more nutrition from the food you eat. In addition, your liver produces bile to help with the absorption of fats. The result of this entire process is that food is reduced to sugars, fatty acids, and amino acids, the fuel for your body.

Here is a summary of enzymes and what they do for your nutrients and how each nutrient is broken down:

> Protease: breaks down protein
>
> Amylase: breaks down starch
>
> Lipase: breaks down fat
>
> Cellulase: breaks down fiber
>
> Lactase: Breaks down lactose (milk sugar)
>
> Papain and Bromelain: primarily protein-digesting enzymes

All raw fruits and vegetables have enzymes; however, some have more than others. Any raw food that has been pasteurized or has preservatives added to them no longer has enzymes, as the enzymes are killed by heat and preservatives. The food will still have nutrients, yet in order to get the full effects of your nutrients, you must have enzymes present. Enzymes help aid absorption and help assure that you receive all the nutrients that you need, thereby resulting in quality health. According to the World's Healthiest Foods Web site, there are more than 2,500 enzymes in food that help with digestion and act as antioxidants.

Bromelain is found in pineapple.

Papain is found in papaya.

Catalase is an antioxidant enzyme found in young sprouts.

Glutahione peroxidase is found in asparagus.

Protease enzyme, papain, as well as chmyopain are found in papaya.

Papain and chymopapain are found in oranges.

Betain, amylase, and maltase are found in beets.

Lipase is found in avocado and coconut.

Maltase is found in bananas, green plants, and beets.

How important are enzymes? Enzymes help to digest proteins, carbohydrates, and fats within the food in the bloodstream. Enzymes help to dramatically improve digestion. Enzymes are proteins used by the body to increase or decrease the speed of chemical reactions. There are many reasons to have raw, natural enzymes in your system, mainly to help your body to function at the greatest peak stability—perfect health.

Some functions of enzymes:

To gain relief from many digestive disorders

Enzymes improve general health and quality of life

Enzymes decrease or eliminate indigestion, gas, bloating, and reflux

Enzymes enhance the body's digestive efficiency, reduce fatigue, and increase your body energy.

Enzymes increase the nutrients you absorb from your diet to improve overall nutrition

Enzymes strengthen the immune system and regenerate cells and tissues.

Enzymes ease stress on digestive organs, especially the pancreas, by reducing their workload.

I believe that the lack of enzymes is one of the paramount causes of premature aging and early death. I also believe it's the underlying cause of almost all degenerative disease. Enzymes are the key to longevity and youthfulness.

Syndromes Common to Enzyme Deficiency

Amylase Deficiency:

- Breaking out of the skin—rash

- Hypoglycemia

- Depression

- PMS

- Hot Flashes

- Fatigue

- Cold hands and feet

- Neck and shoulder aches

- Spruce

- Inflammation

Protease Deficiency:

- Back weakness

- Fungal forms

- Constipation

- High blood pressure

- Insomnia

- Hearing problems

- Parasites

- Gum disorders

- Gingivitis

Lipase Deficiency:

- Aching feet

- Arthritis

- Bladder problems

- Cystitis

- Acne

- Gall bladder stress

- Gallstones

- Hay fever

- Prostate problems

- Psoriasis

Combination Deficiency:

- Chronic allergies

- Common colds

- Diverticulitis

- Irritable bowel syndrome

- Sinus infection

- Immune depressed condition

Foods High in Enzymes

Fruit:

- Avocado
- Banana
- Cantaloupe
- Dates
- Figs
- Grapes
- Guava
- Kiwi
- Mangos
- Melons
- Papaya
- Pineapple

Cultured Foods:

- Cheese
- Kefir
- Yogurt
- Other cultured dairy products
- Butter milk

- Pickle eggs

- Raw sauerkraut

- Raw pickled vegetables

- Pickled beets

- Pickles

- Natto

- Miso

- Soy sauce (traditionally made)

- Tempeh

Other Foods:

- Cucumbers

- Ginger root

- Raw milk

- Raw butter

- Raw honey

- Coconuts

- Germinated tree nuts

- Sprouts

- Wheatgrass juice

- Raw wheat germ

- Flaxseed

- Olive oil

- Olives

- Unrefined oils

The force that enzymes provide is involved in all functions of the body from basic movement, to the function of our organs to the thoughts that come out of our brain. Without enzymes, we cannot move, feel, hear, see, or, think. No living thing can exist without enzymes. All cells in our body depend upon enzymes for function. Life cannot exist without enzymes. Enzymes are the key factor that determines the effectiveness of how your body functions.

We are born with trillions of these mysterious life forces called enzymes. Once they are used up, there is no longer any life. However, if you eat a large amount of raw fruits and vegetables, you can slow down the use of the enzymes. The truth is that you have severely slowed down your metabolism and drained your enzyme bank account by eating a lot of wrong foods and by starving yourself on fad diets.

The importance of enzymes cannot be overstated; enzymes are life itself.

VITAMIN D

Vitamin D is very essential for good health. Vitamin D is essential for the human body to function properly. It regulates over 200 genes in cells all over the body, including the brain, heart, kidney, bone, intestine, skin, gonads, prostate, breast, parathyroid gland, and immune system. The two major forms are vitamin D2 and vitamin D3. Vitamin D2 is found in fungi and plants. Vitamin D3 is synthesized in our skin when it is exposed to Ultraviolet B (UVB) light from the sun. It's also found in fish oil, but the most significant source of vitamin D comes from the interaction of UV light on the skin (United States Department of Agriculture).

Vitamin D is also known as the sunshine vitamin. According to The National Institute Health (NIH), Vitamin D is endogenously made when ultraviolet rays from the sun strike the skin and trigger vitamin D synthesis. The skin should be exposed to mid-morning or early evening sunlight, two to three times a week, as the rays are not as direct and damaging at these times. About ten to fifteen minutes of direct, unprotected sunlight is all it takes for the body to create the amount of vitamin D needed for the day.

A balance is required between the use of sun block to protect the skin from sun damage and yet still allow some UV rays onto the skin in order to achieve sufficient vitamin D production. The skin acts like solar panels; it stores and releases Vitamin D when it is needed by the body. Many factors can make obtaining enough sunshine and thus the production of vitamin D difficult:

Complete cloud cover reduces UV energy by 50 percent

UVB energy does not penetrate glass

Sunscreen with a protection factor of 8 or more blocks UVB light and your ability to manufacture vitamin D (Office of Dietary Supplements)

*Note: this only when you are getting the morning sun, you must use protection when in the sun for long periods of time. Do not over expose!

In actuality, vitamin D is a fat-soluble hormone. When it was first discovered, vitamin D was labeled as a vitamin, but after further research, it was determined to be a hormone. The fact that vitamin D is a hormone could suggest why it can be made by the body. Vitamin D3 synthesis begins in the skin. Then the liver and kidneys process vitamin D to its final active form, calcitriol. Some studies have found that vitamin D3 has longer lasting effects than vitamin D2, while other studies have found them equally effective.

The principal function of vitamin D in all vertebrates, including humans, is to maintain serum calcium and phosphorus concentrations in a range that supports ossification. Vitamin D accomplishes this goal by enhancing the efficiency of the small intestine to absorb dietary calcium and phosphorus and by mobilizing calcium and phosphorus stores from bone. Simply put, it controls the amount of calcium absorption by the intestine and works in conjunction with other minerals and compounds in the bone making/maintaining team.

Vitamin D promotes bone mineralization by making calcium and phosphorous available in the blood and then depositing the minerals in the bone as it hardens. Vitamin D increases the blood concentration of these two minerals by increasing absorption of the minerals from the gastrointestinal tract and by retention from the kidneys. Without vitamin D, only about 10 to 15 percent of dietary calcium and about 60 percent of phosphorus is absorbed by the body. This is directly related to bone mineral density, which is responsible for osteoporosis and fractures, as well as muscle strength and falls in adult. In utero and in childhood, calcium and vitamin D deficiency prevents the maximum deposition of calcium in the skeleton.

Vitamin D is carried in the bloodstream to the liver where it is converted into the prohormone, calcidiol. Circulating calcidiol may then be converted into calcitriol, the biologically active form of vitamin D, in the kidneys. Calcitriol acts locally as a cytokine, defending the body against microbial invaders.

When synthesized in the kidneys, calcitriol circulates as a hormone. It then regulates, among other things, the concentration of calcium and phosphate in the bloodstream, promoting the healthy mineralization, growth, and remodeling of bone, and the prevention of hypocalcemic tetany. Vitamin D insufficiency can result in thin, brittle or misshapen bones, while sufficiency prevents rickets in children and osteomalacia in adults, and together with calcium, helps to protect older adults from osteoporosis. Vitamin D also modulates neuromuscular function, reduces inflammation, and influences that action of many genes that regulate the proliferation, differentiation, and apoptosis (death) of cells.

Because it regulates calcium and phosphorus levels in the blood, vitamin D can suppress the immune system and help to fight against conditions like rheumatoid arthritis, lupus, and multiple sclerosis. Vitamin D can activate the immune system to fight cancer and infections like tuberculosis, pneumonia, and flu and decrease the risk of heart attacks and strokes. Vitamin D helps prevent diabetes by modifying the release and response to insulin.

Do not underestimate the importance of this hormone. The more I study, the more that I see how so much sickness and disease is possibly connected to not having this vitamin/hormone in our diet. This hormone controls many aspects that have to do with vital health. It seems to control everything from weight control to our hormones and good health.

Natural Food Sources of Vitamin D:

- Fatty fish species

- Catfish

- Salmon, cooked

- Mackerel, cooked

- Sardines, canned in oil drained

- Tuna, canned in oil

- Eel, cooked

- Whole eggs

- Beef liver, cooked

- Fish liver oils, such as cod liver oil

- Mushrooms

ANTIOXIDANTS

Antioxidants are compounds that help protect the body's immune system. They are found naturally in fruits and vegetables and are added to foods and skin care products. Antioxidants keep us healthy. They are extremely important because they are compounds that help protect the body against problems created by stress, poor diet, and environmental pollutants.

It is important to understand antioxidants, and it is important to understand oxidative stress and free radicals. Oxidative stress is the effect of oxidation where unstable molecules, such as free radicals, lead to cellular damage. The molecules are considered unstable because they are missing a component such as oxygen. Antioxidants give the free radicals the oxygen molecule that is missing, thus making them stable. Free radicals are atoms or groups of atoms with an odd (unpaired) number of electrons and can be formed when oxygen interacts with certain molecules.

When the cells in our body use oxygen, they naturally produce free radicals as by-products, which can cause cellular damage. Free radicals can damage your

DNA. This is why it is so important to control the free radicals in the body. Antioxidants are compounds that help protect our bodies from the abundance of free radicals. Antioxidants are molecules that can safely interact with free radicals and terminate the chain reaction before vital molecules are damaged. Antioxidants are dietary compounds such as vitamins, minerals, amino acids, and phytonutrients that directly bind to and destroy damaging free radicals, which can prevent or slow the oxidative damage to our body.

Free radicals form in the body in response to stress, poor diet, aging, smoking, toxins, and pollutants in the air we breathe. Stress can be mental or physical, and even exercising can increase the free radical formation. Once formed, these highly reactive radicals can start a chain reaction, like dominoes. As metabolites or products of oxidation reactions, free radicals can negatively impact the structure and function of the body. The chief danger of free radicals comes from damage they can do when they react with important cellular components, such as DNA or the cell membrane. If the free radicals react with DNA or cell membranes, cells may loss function and die. To prevent free radical damage, the body has a defense system of antioxidants. Antioxidants act as free radical scavengers and, hence, prevent and repair damage done by free radicals.

Sometimes free radicals are beneficial. In desired amounts, they can help fight infections and decrease the amount of cancer cells. They start to harm the body when they get out of control by multiplying or occurring in large amounts. The abundance of free radicals can lead to several health issues like atherosclerosis, osteoarthritis, hepatitis, cirrhosis of the liver, immune deviancies, cancer, premature aging, and other problems.

The effectiveness of any given antioxidant in the body depends on which free radical is involved, how/where it is generated, and location of the damage. While in one particular system, an antioxidant may protect against free radicals, in other systems it could have no effect at all. Or in certain circumstances, like with copper, an antioxidant may even act as a pro-oxidant and generates toxic oxygen species. This is why it is important to have balance. Antioxidants themselves become oxidized, which is why there is a constant need to replenish our antioxidant resources.

Antioxidant Classification

Chain breaking: When a free radical releases or steals an electron, a second radical is formed. This molecule then turns around and does the same thing to a third molecule, continuing to generate more unstable products. The process continues until termination occurs. Either the radical is stabilized by a chain-breaking antioxidant such as beta-carotene and vitamins C and E, or it simply decays into harmless product.

Preventive: Antioxidant enzymes can prevent oxidation by reducing the rate of chain initiation. This prevention occurs by scavenging for the initiating radicals. These antioxidants can thwart an oxidation chain from ever being set into motion. They can also prevent oxidization by stabilizing transition metal radicals such as copper and iron.

Antioxidants List:

- Vitamins: A, C, E

- Minerals: Zinc, Copper, Selenium, Magnesium

- Beta-carotene

- Enzyme systems

Rather than work alone, antioxidant vitamins and minerals work together in synergy as each antioxidant depends upon another to help support its optimal function. Antioxidants should be used as a team rather than by themselves. A combination of antioxidants is more effective than a single antioxidant. The mineral selenium with vitamin E is a great antioxidant combination. Vitamin C and beta-carotene are also excellent antioxidants. When the immune function is damaged by free radicals, a team of antioxidants is needed to help fight off the free radicals and give the immune system a boost. For example, a team of schizandra berries, vitamins C and E, beta-carotene, and the mineral selenium will help protect the cells of the body.

Although there are several enzyme systems within the body that scavenge free radicals, the principle micronutrient (vitamin) antioxidants are vitamin E, beta-carotene, and vitamin C. Additionally, selenium, a trace mineral, is required for proper function of one of the body's antioxidant enzyme system and is sometimes included in this category. The body cannot manufacture these micronutrients, so they must be supplied in the diet.

Phytonutrients are plant-based nutrients that have power antioxidants. There is a wide range of reasons as why to eat a variety of colors from the produce aisle. Among the fact that fruits and vegetables are relatively fat free and a great means of getting fiber, they also have phytonutrients, which we need to help protect our bodies. Carrots and cantaloupes are a great source of vitamin A. Vitamin A helps maintain eye health and with the body's immunity. Bananas and spinach are a source of potassium that is necessary for proper nerve and muscle function. Broccoli and asparagus are excellent sources of the B vitamins that help convert food into energy. Phytonutrients are contained in all fruits and vegetables and can help protect the body's vital organs, which include the eyes, heart, lungs, liver, skin, etc.

Antioxidant Food Sources

Vitamin A: brightly colored fruits and vegetables like carrots, squash, sweet potatoes, tomatoes, cantaloupe, peaches, apricots, watermelon, kiwi, oranges, blackberries; green leafy vegetables like kale, collards, broccoli, spinach, peas, green peepers, asparagus, avocado, pumpkin seeds, pine nuts, almonds, sunflower seeds, pistachios, chestnuts

Vitamin C: citrus fruits like oranges, lime, and lemon; green peppers; broccoli; green leafy vegetables like spinach and kale; strawberries; tomatoes; peach; apples; grapes; artichoke; asparagus; avocado; broccoli; carrots; cauliflower; corn; cucumber; lima beans; mushrooms; onions; peas; potatoes; squash; sweet potato

Vitamin E: nuts and seeds, i.e. almonds, sunflower seeds, pine nuts, peanuts, brazil nuts; whole grains, green leafy vegetables, vegetable oil and liver; blackberries; bananas; apples; kiwi; mango; apple

Selenium: fish and shellfish, red meat, grains, eggs, chicken, and garlic. Kiwi fruit, tomatoes, blackberries, bananas, strawberry, orange, peach, lime, cantaloupe, lima beans, peas, artichoke, avocado, corn, potatoes, asparagus, broccoli, kale, mushrooms, sweet potato, sunflower seeds, brazil nuts, cashews, pine nuts, pistachios, almonds, walnuts, chestnuts, pecans, macadamias, hazelnuts, and pumpkin seeds

Copper: organ meats, seafood, nuts, seeds, wheat bran, cereals, whole grain products, cocoa products. Most fruits contain a small amount, such as kiwi fruit, apples, bananas, blackberries, cantaloupe, grapes, lemon, lime, orange, peach, strawberry, and tomatoes.

Magnesium: green leafy vegetables, spinach, potatoes, nuts, seeds, whole grain, including bran, wheat oats, and chocolate. Smaller amounts are found in many foods including bananas, broccoli, raisins, and shrimp.

Zinc: red meat, poultry, some seafood, whole grains, dry beans, and nuts. Most vegetables have zinc. Blackberries, kiwi, peas, lima beans, squash, potatoes, corn, sweet potato, pumpkin seeds, pine nuts, cashews, sunflower seeds, pecans, Brazil nuts, almonds, walnuts

PHYTONUTRIENTS

We have all heard that it is important to eat fruits and vegetables every day. Some of us actually do eat the minimum recommended servings. Science has now discovered that consuming increased amounts of fruits and vegetables can provide even greater health benefits.

The value of fruits and vegetables goes beyond that of the vitamins and minerals that they contain; it is the discovery of a class of micronutrients. These micronutrients called "phytonutrients" or "phytochemicals" are largely why major health agencies recommended a minimum of five different fruits and vegetables daily. Dr. John H Maher, ABAAHP states that phytonutrients appear to be essential for optimal health and longevity and therefore may properly be classed as micronutrients, along with vitamins and minerals.

Phytochemicals are compounds that exist in plants to protect them from the sunlight that are neither vitamin nor mineral and affect human beings and other mammals in a number of beneficial ways. The more phytochemicals you add to your diet, the greater the degree of health protection you can enjoy. They have tremendous health benefits and are available in thousands of our foods. Phytonutrients have anti-inflammatory benefits, help our cells communicate with one another, and can help prevent facilitating cancer cells. People who eat large quantities of fruits and vegetables have reduced risks of cancer. A lifelong diet of phytochemical plays an important role in health longevity.

Our bodies need oxygen to live, and the result of the use of oxygen is a process known as oxidation. Just like any metal will rust (oxidation), our bodies go through a similar process over time. Phytonutrients act as antioxidants that help keep our cells from oxidation. Phytonutrients protects us from diseases such as cancer, diabetes, heart disease, and arthritis. The American diet is sorely lacking in these nutrients. By eating more color fruits, vegetables, whole grains, nuts, and seeds, we would go a long way to improving our health and eliminating chronic diseases.

The beneficial phytonutrients are:

Polyhenols are antioxidants that act as an anti-inflammatory. Foods such as nuts, berries, and teas contain this phytonutrient.

Phytosterols help with the inhibition of cholesterol absorption, modulation of hormone metabolism, immune function, and inflammatory physiology. Nuts are the richest source of phytosterols. Numerous studies demonstrate that diets rich in nuts and seeds are associated with a decreased occurrence of cardiovascular disease (CVD).

Carotenoids are a variety of pigments in our foods that give them their red and yellow appearance. This group of phytonutrients contains beta-carotene, lutein, and lycopene. They are found in our fruits and vegetables such as tomatoes, carrots, pumpkin, apricots, and sweet potatoes. There is some evidence that they help protect us from cancer and have anti-aging properties. Lutein and lycopene require fat for optimal uptake of carotenoids, whereas dietary fiber inhibits its absorption of lutein, lycopene, and beta-carotene by 40 to 75 percent.

Beta-carotene intake is associated with reduced risk of breast, stomach, esophageal, and pancreatic cancers. Fourteen researchers from John Hopkins reported in 1994 that smokers with the lowest blood levels of beta-carotene had approximately a 350 percent greater risk of heart attack as compared to non-smokers with high beta-carotene levels. To my surprise, Dr. Maher said that some carotenoid-rich foods like carrots and tomatoes yield more beta-carotene and lycopene, respectively, when *cooked*.

Remember our bodies benefit from a rich infusion of these nutrients. When it comes to fighting cancer, cruciferous vegetables may be the team champs. These plant micronutrients work by speeding up the production of enzymes, especially in the liver, with which our bodies convert toxic, mutagenic (cancer causing) chemicals into less harmful substances. *The Journal of the National Cancer Institute* proclaimed that cruciferous vegetables substantially lowered the risk of prostate cancer in men. Various studies also suggest a protective role in cervical, uterine, and breast cancers in women. It is important to know which fruits and vegetables contain these important phytochemicals.

The National Cancer Institute recognizes the following twelve fruits and vegetables important for their phytonutrient content:

- pineapple
- papaya
- turnips
- carrots
- tomatoes
- cauliflower
- cabbage
- kale
- Brussels sprouts
- broccoli
- garlic
- onions

So to sum it all up, to change your life for good health, longevity, and a quality of life, eat plenty of raw fruits, vegetables, whole grains, legumes, and nuts because of the phytonutrients they contain.

ESSENTIAL AMINO ACIDS

Essential amino acids are necessary for good health but cannot be produced by the body. Essential amino acids must be found in diet. There are nine amino acids generally considered essential for humans. The essential amino acids are histidine, leucine, isoleucine, lysine, methionine, phenylalanine, theorine, valine, and tryptophan. All essential amino acids can be found in vegetables.

Amino acids have a profound effect on how we feel, how clearly we think, and the physical constitution of our bodies. Even non-essential amino acids produced within our bodies require the right combination of supporting nutrients for the most favorable protein maintenance. A healthy diet should always be sustained.

Histidine (used in the treatment of rheumatoid arthritis):

- May boost T-cell function, which helps with auto-immune disease, such as HIV and AIDS

- Important for the maintenance of the myelin sheaths that protect the nerve cells. (Any shaking-type disease would benefit.)

- May help with nerve deafness

- Helps with sexual arousal

- May help with indigestion due to lack of stomach acid

- Needed for the production of both red and white the blood cells

- Protects the body from irradiation

- Aids in removing heavy metals from the system

Food Sources: rice, wheat, rye

Leucine:

- Slows muscle degradation by facilitating the creation of muscle proteins

- Used by the liver, body fat, and muscle

- Increases energy and endurance

- Also plays an important role in the synthesis of hemoglobin

- Maintains proper blood sugar and plays a role in human growth hormone synthesis

Food Sources: soybeans; mature, raw seeds; lentils; cow peas; beef peanuts; salami; Italian pork; fish; pink salmon; raw nuts; almonds; flax seed; walnuts; English asparagus

Isoleucine:

- Used for hemoglobin formation

- Stabilizes and regulates blood sugar levels

- Used to enhance energy, increase endurance, and aid in healing and repair of muscle tissue

- Used for mental disorders

- Deficiency may look like hypoglycemia

Food Sources: almonds, cashews, chicken, chickpeas (garbanzo beans), eggs, fish, lentils, liver, meat, rye, most seed and soy protein.

Lysine:

- Helps maintain proper nitrogen balance

- Inhibits herpes (works best when you minimize arginine intake)

- Assists building muscle mass, collagen formation, and tissue repair

- Good for those recovering from surgery and sports injuries

- Helps lower high serum triglycerides

- Helps prevent fertility problems

- Improves concentration

- Important for proper bone and growth development in children

- Used in the production of antibodies, hormones, and enzymes

- Helps with calcium absorption

Food Sources: fish, eggs, milk, lima beans, meat, cheese, potatoes, soy products, yeast, and most proteins.

Methionine:

- Supplies sulfur to the body

- Used for the treatment of AIDS patients

- May improve memory recall in cases with nervous system degeneration

- May help with Parkinson's disease

- Used in the treatment of pancreatitis

- Used to support liver function

- Low intake of methionine during pregnancy is associated with neural tube defects

- May help to prevent the clogging of arteries by eliminating plaque

- Assists in the breakdown of fats

- Helps detoxify lead and other heavy metals

- Helps to prevent brittle hair

- Protects against radiation

- Beneficial for those with osteoporosis

- Helps with chemical allergies, rheumatic fever, and pregnancy toxemia

- Powerful antioxidant that inactivates free radicals

- Promotes the excretion of estrogen

Food Sources: meat, liver, dairy, garlic, lentils, onions, soybeans, seeds, yogurt

Phenylalanine:

- Used for depression (phenylalanine is converted to tyrosine, which in turn synthesizes dopamine and norepinephrine)

- Used for alcohol withdraw support

- Used for osteoarthritis and rheumatoid arthritis

- Used for vertigo

- Potential mood elevator

- May help control addictive behavior

- Promotes sexual arousal

- Reduces hunger and cravings for food

- DL-Phenylalanine form may influence the brain and its way of dealing with pain relief by stimulating endorphins. Its painkilling response increases over time.

- Used for menstrual cramps, migraines, and other pain

- May be helpful with Parkinson's

- Used for migraine pain, neuralgia and leg cramps

Food Sources: proteins, cheese, almonds, peanuts, soybeans

Theronine:

- Maintains proper protein balance in the body

- Important in the formation of collagen and elastin

- Aids liver and lipotrophic function

- Helps prevent fatty buildup in the liver

- Enhances immune system by aiding in the production of antibodies

Food Sources: fish, beef, soy, wheat, brown rice, bread, liver, peanuts (raw)

Tryptophan:

- Necessary for the production of B3 (niacin) in the body

- Used by the brain to produce serotonin

- Responsible for normal sleep

- Helps combat depression and insomnia

- Stabilizes mood

- Helps control hyperactivity in children

- Alleviates stress

- Good for the heart

- Aids in weight control by decreasing appetite

- Good for migraine headaches

- May reduce some effects of nicotine

- Deficiency may lead to coronary artery spasm

- Helps decrease sensitivity to pain

- May help fibromyalgia and migraines

Food Sources: brown rice, cottage cheese, meat, peanuts, soy protein

Valine:

- Has a stimulant effect

- Needed for muscle metabolism and tissue repair

- Necessary for proper nitrogen balance in the body

- Can be used as an energy source by muscles

- Corrects severe amino deficiencies caused by drug addictions

- Too much may lead to feelings of skin crawling

Food sources: dairy, grains, meat, mushrooms, peanuts, soy protein

PROBIOTICS

The term probiotic literally means "for life" in Greek, and it refers to bacteria. Probiotics are live microorganisms—in most cases, bacteria—that are similar to beneficial microorganisms normally found in the human intestinal tract. Probiotics play a vital role in the fermentation and digestion of carbohydrates and aid in the digestion of fats and proteins.

It has been estimated that more microbial cells exist in the human body than human cells. Out of the many hundreds of kinds of bacteria that live inside your body, many of them are in your gut. These bacteria include many different microbes, both good and bad, which help to maintain the natural balance of organisms in the intestines. Most of the bacteria in the human system are good bacteria. Microorganisms are collectively called your gut flora, micro flora, or beneficial bacteria and are estimated to make up about three pounds of your body weight. They are essential to keep you alive.

Digestive microbes are a natural part of the human nutrition system, as humans cannot produce all of the nutrients we need. Gut flora can digest carbohydrates that humans would not be able to digest otherwise, and they also produce biotin and vitamin K. Probiotics are also referred to as friendly/good bacteria. Probiotics are especially in the intestinal tract of breastfed infants who have been provided this natural protection against diseases by their mothers.

Friendly bacteria are vital to proper development of the immune system, to protect against microorganisms that could cause disease, and to the digestion and absorption of food and nutrients. Each person's mix of bacteria varies. Interactions between a person and the microorganisms in their body and among the microorganisms themselves can be crucial to the person's health and well being.

According to the World Health Organization and the Food and Agriculture Organization of the United Nations, probiotics administered in adequate amounts confer a health benefit on the host. Probiotics are available to consumers mainly in the form of foods and can be used as a form of complementary and alternative medicine.

Scientific understanding of probiotics and their potential for preventing and treating health conditions is at an early stage but moving ahead. In November 2005, in a conference that was cofounded by the National Center for Complementary and Alternative Medicine (NCCAM) America Society for Microbiology, the topic of probiotic use was explored. A Stanford study seems to indicate that weight gain could be the result of a bacterial infection. When probiotics or the good bacteria populate the digestive system, the bad bacteria start to move out. Another part of the interest in probiotics stems from the fact there are cells in the digestive tract connected with the immune system. One theory is that if you alter the microorganisms in a person's intestinal tract (as by introducing probiotic bacteria), you can affect the immune system's defenses.

The bacterial balancing act can be thrown off in two major ways:

1.   Antibiotics: They kill friendly bacteria in the gut along with unfriendly bacteria. Some people use probiotics to try to offset side effects from antibiotics like gas, cramping, or diarrhea. Similarly, some use them to ease symptoms of lactose intolerance, a condition in which the gut lacks the enzyme needed to digest significant amounts of the major sugar in milk and also causes gastrointestinal symptoms.

2.   Unfriendly microorganisms: These organisms—bacteria, yeasts, fungi, and parasites—can cause disease, which can upset the internal balance. Researchers are exploring whether probiotics could halt these unfriendly agents in the first place and/or suppress their growth and activity in conditions like:

- Irritable bowel syndrome

- Inflammatory bowel disease (e.g. ulcerative colitis and Crohn's disease)

- Infection with helicobacter pylori (H. pylori), bacterium that causes most ulcers and many types of chronic stomach inflammation

- Tooth decay and periodontal disease

- Vaginal infections

- Stomach and respiratory infections that children acquire in daycare

- Skin infections

When we eat over-processed foods, they kill the good microbes. It is like when you cook foods; the heating process kills microbes. It is good to kill the bad microbes in our food in order to avoid sickness and disease. However, this process works just like chemotherapy, which kills the bad cells as well as the good. Since you kill the good bacteria, you must replace good microbes with nutrients from food: raw fruit and vegetables and fermented foods. It is important to have a healthy balance of beneficial microbes to avoid sickness and disease in order to keep your body nutritionally sound.

Things that can destroy our good probiotics:

- Antibiotic use

- Too much alcohol

- The over consumption of sugars and other refined carbohydrates

- The distress of too much stress

- The lack of nutrition from living fresh foods grown in nutrient-rich soil

- Drinking chlorinated water destroys our intestinal flora. The reason we put chlorine in the water is because it is able to kill bacteria and unfortunately, it gets the good ones along with the bad when we drink it.

- The medical treatment of radiation and chemotherapy also destroys our intestinal flora as well as damaging our immune systems. Any course of chemotherapy should be followed with heavy doses of probiotics.

- Alcoholic beverages tend to harm probiotics by killing them directly and encourage harmful bacteria and yeast overgrowth.

Probiotic Food Sources:

- Fermented foods

- Sauerkraut

- Dill pickles

- Miso

- Tempeh

- A beverage called *RyWhe*

- Raw fruits and vegetables

I personally believe that the reason we have so much sickness and disease is because we kill off all the good bacteria in the gut by eating highly processed foods, refined sugars, refined flour, high fructose corn syrup, and foods that are filled with preservatives and foods that have been depleted of all of their nutrients. I am convinced that, by eating lots of raw fruits and vegetables and eating less processed and refined food, you can create a catalysis in your body and reach better health.

MINERALS

Minerals are vital for life. Yet, despite their importance, the human body is not equipped to produce the minerals it needs to function. These nutrients must be obtained from food. Minerals are required by the body in relatively small amounts. It is important to make sure your diet provides minerals, as the absence of these minerals can lead to illness and disease.

Minerals and trace minerals have a tremendous impact on the body, and when these minerals become deficient for whatever reason, it can cause your body to do a total tailspin. Minerals are as important to the human body as breathing; without the proper amount of minerals, our body would cease to function properly. If the deficiency is severe enough, it can and will result in death.

Minerals have an effect on nearly every single function in the body. One of these key actions is to act as a reactor to many essential vitamins and nutrients. In other words, you can take vitamins every day, but if you are not taking the correct minerals to bind with the vitamins, they will simply get excreted and not be used properly by the body. Minerals must be absorbed by the body before they can be used effectively. Your body needs minerals each day, and these can generally be supplied by eating a balanced diet.

Minerals are classified into two groups: major minerals and trace minerals. Major minerals are required by the body in larger amounts. Trace minerals are required in smaller amounts yet are still needed for quality health.

The major minerals that are required by the body are: calcium, magnesium, sodium, potassium, chloride, and phosphorus,

Calcium is important for building and maintaining strong bones and teeth, muscle contraction, and blood clotting. It is found in dairy products, leafy green vegetables, almonds, sesame seeds, and dried fruit pulses.

Magnesium supports bone mineralization, enzyme activation, protein building, muscle contractions (including the heart), nerve impulse transmission, immunity, and bone and teeth formation. Magnesium is found in plant foods, such as spinach, broccoli, artichokes, parsley, spinach, broccoli, green beans, tomato juice, navy beans, pinto beans, black-eyed peas, sunflower seeds, tofu, cashews, and halibut.

Sodium maintains fluid and electrolyte balance and supports muscle contractions and nerve impulse transmissions. It is found in: salt, soy sauce, bread, milk, and meats.

Potassium also maintains fluid and electrolyte balance. It maintains cell integrity, muscle contractions, and nerve impulse transmission. Potassium is found in potatoes, acorn, squash, artichoke, spinach, broccoli, carrots, green beans, tomato juice, avocado, grapefruit juice, watermelon, bananas, strawberries, cod, and milk.

Phosphorus is required along with calcium for strong bones, teeth, and muscle function. It is a vital component of all body cells and found in nearly all foods.

Chloride maintains fluid and electrolyte balance and aids in digestion. It is found in many vegetables including celery and tomatoes, milk, eggs, meats.

Sulphur is used in the formation of amino acids, hormones, connective tissues, and carbohydrate metabolism. Found in beans sprouts, leafy green vegetables, raspberries, dairy products, red meat, egg yolk, chicken, seafood, legumes, and nuts.

Trace Minerals: Iron, zinc, chromium, copper, fluoride, selenium, iodine, and molybdenum

Iron is an essential component of hemoglobin. Hemoglobin transports oxygen in the blood through the body. Found in leafy green vegetables, pulses, whole bread, dried fruit, pumpkin seeds, and molasses. Vitamin C helps to absorb iron. Caffeine can reduce the amount of iron absorbed.

Zinc is a part of many enzymes involved in production of genetic material and proteins and helps to transport vitamin A. Zinc is also important for taste perception, wound healing, sperm production, and normal development of the fetus. It is found in: spinach, broccoli, green peas, green beans, tomato juice, lentils, oysters, shrimp, crab, turkey (dark meat), lean ham, lean ground beef, lean sirloin steak, plain yogurt, Swiss cheese, tofu, ricotta cheese.

Chromium is associated with insulin and is required for the release of energy from glucose (blood glucose control). It is found in: vegetable oils, liver, brewer's yeast, whole grains, cheese, nuts, potato, broccoli, green beans, tomato, apples, banana, grapes, oranges, red meat, turkey.

Copper helps your body utilize iron and is useful in red blood cell formation; healthy bones and teeth; heart and nervous system function; and skin, hair, and eye pigmentation. Food sources: turnip greens, molasses, chard, spinach, kale, mustard greens, asparagus, eggplant, peppermint, tomatoes, ginger, tempeh, sesame seeds, and sunflower seeds.

Fluoride is important for the resistance to tooth decay and is found in seafood.

Selenium is an antioxidant that works with vitamin E, protects cells from damage, immune and thyroid function. It is found in fish, shellfish, poultry, brazil nuts, brown rice, wheat-germ, and whole meal bread.

Iodine is a component of thyroid hormones that help regulate growth, development, and metabolic rate. It is found in sea salt, seafood, bread, milk, and cheese.

Molybdenum facilitates many cell processes. It is found in legumes and organ meats.

VITAMINS

Vitamins are a group of food substance or nutrients found only in living things, such as plants and animals. They can also be defined as complex chemical substances contained mainly in foods required for normal growth. Most vitamins cannot be made in your body, so they must be acquired from food.

Vitamins have no calories and no energy source; however, they do assist in metabolizing nutrients in food and are invaluable in keeping your body running smoothly. Vitamins enable the body to break down and use the basic elements of food: proteins, carbohydrates, and fats. They also make it possible for other nutrients to be digested, absorbed, and metabolized by the body. The excess or lack of vitamins can lead to acute and chronic disease. Certain vitamins are also involved in producing blood cells, hormones, and genetic material in chemicals in your nervous system.

Vitamins mainly serve as catalysts for certain reactions in the body, as they combine with proteins to create metabolically active enzymes. These enzymes in turn produce hundreds of important chemical reactions throughout the body. The fundamentals of cells depend greatly upon vitamins. Without vitamins, our cells would not function properly, and thus, our organs would suffer and eventually we would no longer be able to survive.

List Of Vitamins:

- Vitamin A (retinol)

- Vitamin B1 (thiamine)

- Vitamin B2 (riboflavin)

- Vitamin B3 (niacin)

- Vitamin B5 (pantothenic acid, pantothenate)

- Vitamin B6 (pyridoxine)

- Vitamin B7 (biotin)

- Vitamin B9 (folate, folacin, folic acid)

- Vitamin B12 (cobalamin)

- Vitamin C (ascorbic acid)

- Vitamin D (1,25 dihydroxycholicalciferol)

- Vitamin E (tocopherol)

- Vitamin K

An enzyme is a protein, while a coenzyme is a vitamin, mineral, or other small molecule. A coenzyme is a small molecule that combines with an enzyme to make it active. Vitamins do not provide energy, but vitamins

B1, B2, and B3 work as coenzymes to convert energy nutrients into energy the body can use. Bacteria present in the gut, called human flora, make vitamin K, biotin, and choline. Choline is a B-complex vitamin that is a constituent of lecithin essential in the metabolism of fat.

Precursors or provitamins are compounds that can be converted into active vitamins in the body. It is more accurate to count both the active form and the available value of the vitamin from the precursor. Some vitamins like niacin, vitamin A, and vitamin D have precursors. Vitamins are very important because they perform various functions in our body.

Vitamin Classes

Vitamins are separated into two classes based on their solubility. Solubility imparts many characteristic behaviors to vitamins and determines how they are absorbed and transported around the blood stream, how they are stored in the body, and how easily they excreted from the body. The classes are fat-soluble and water-soluble vitamins.

Fat Soluble vitamins contain carbon, hydrogen, and oxygen and can be dissolved in lipids (fat-like substances). Fat-soluble vitamins can be stored in appreciable amounts in the body with other lipids in the fatty tissues. Because these vitamins can be stored, they may be toxic in excessive amounts. They travel in blood associated with protein carriers. They require bile for absorption and are absorbed from the intestines into the lymphatic system.

- Vitamin A (retinol)- Beta carotene is provitamin A

- Vitamin D (1,25 dihydroxycholicalciferol)

- Vitamin E (tocopherol)

- Vitamin K (phylloquinone, menaquinone)

Water-soluble vitamins contain carbon, hydrogen, oxygen, and nitrogen and sometimes sulfur. These vitamins are absorbed directly into the blood stream and travel freely in blood. The water-soluble vitamins cannot be stored in the body or tissues to any great extent. The excess is excreted in the urine, therefore making the risk of toxicity small.

- Vitamin B1 (thiamine)

- Vitamin B2 (riboflavin)

- Vitamin B3 (niacin)

- Vitamin B5 (pantothenic acid, pantothenate)

- Vitamin B6 (pyridoxine)

- Vitamin B7 (biotin)

- Vitamin B9 (folate, folacin, folic acid)

- Vitamin B12 (cyanocobalamin)

- Vitamin C

Functions of Vitamins:

- Responsible for keeping cells strong

- Fight infections, ensure protection against viruses

- Regulate metabolism, and good health

- Help convert fat and carbohydrates into energy

- Assist in forming bone and tissue

- Important for proper growth of children

- Help hormone formation

- Help with blood cells formation

- Assist in formation of nervous system chemicals and genetic material

Vitamins are essential, which means we must get them from food because the body cannot make them. An adequate intake of vitamins protects against deficiency diseases and reduces the risk of a number of chronic diseases. Each vitamin has a range of intake in which it functions optimally. Eating five or more servings of fruits and vegetables is a good way to get enough vitamins in the diet each day. Consumption below or above these ranges impairs health.

Fat Soluble

Vitamin A:
  Functions:

- Formation of mucous membrane and maintenance of skin and bone

- For vision in dim light

- Beta-carotene acts as antioxidant to cell membranes and is the precursor or provitamin of Vitamin A

Deficiencies:

- Susceptibility to infections including measles and HIV

- Impaired vision, inability to see in dim light

- Keratinization, the condition when keratin (an insoluble protein) accumulates in the cornea

- Causes xerophthalmia, condition where vitamin A deficiency causes drying and thickening of the eye

- It is a leading cause of blindness in developing countries

*Note: you cannot overdose on the precurosor to vitamin A, beta-carotene. The body converts beta-carotene plus other carotenes present into vitamin A.

Vitamin D: Vitamin D is manufactured from cholesterol in cells under the skin with exposure to sunlight. In actuality, vitamin D is a hormone, but more about that later.

Functions:

Needed for the absorption of calcium and phosphorus in the intestines and bones.

Deficiencies:

- In children: weak, deformed bones, a disease called rickets

- In adults: lost of calcium from bones, a disease called osteoporosis

Vitamin E (tocopherol): Oils naturally contain Vitamin E as an antioxidant.
Functions:
Antioxidant

- prevents damage to cell membranes in blood cells, lungs and other tissues by repairing the damage

- May reduce the ability of LDL (bad cholesterol) to form plaque in arteries

Deficiencies:

- Muscle loss, nerve damage

- Anemia and weakness

Vitamin K: It is produced in the intestines by bacteria. Vitamin K injections are given to newborns because they do not have bacteria in their intestine.
Functions:

- Essential component of blood clotting system

- Aids in calcium incorporation in bones

Deficiencies:

- Bleeding, bruises

- Decreased calcium in bones

- Deficiency is rare, but long term use of antibiotics can cause deficiency

Water Soluble

Vitamin B1—Thiamin:
Functions:

- All cells use thiamin to help the body to release energy from carbohydrates

- Helps growth and maintains nerves and muscles

- Promotes normal appetite

Deficiencies:

- (beriberi)

- Fatigue, weakness

- Nerve disorders, mental confusion and apathy

- Heart irregularity and failure

Vitamin B3—Niacin
Functions:

- Helps body capture and use energy released from carbohydrates, proteins, and fats

- Assists in the manufacture of body fats

- Helps maintain normal nervous system functions

Deficiencies:

- (pellagra)

- Skin disorders

- Nervous and mental disorders

- Diarrhea, indigestion

- Fatigue

Vitamin B7—Biotin
Functions:

- Supports healthy skin through proper fat production

- Helps your body make efficient use of support

- Maintains an energy supply

- Helps transfer carbon dioxide

- Helps maintain a steady blood sugar level

- Recommended for strengthening hair and nails

- Biotin helps move sugar from its initial stages of processing to its conversion into usable chemical energy

Deficiencies:

- Depression neurological symptoms, such as depression hallucination lethargy, nervousness and numbness tingling of the extremities

- Hair loss

- Conjunctivitis (eye infections)

- Dermatitis: in the form of scaly red rash around the eyes, nose, mouth, and genital area

- Impaired immune system function

- Fungal infections

Vitamin B9—Folate, Folic Acid
Functions:

- Needed for reactions that utilize amino acids for protein tissue formation

- Needed for the DNA of new cells, therefore is required for formation of all new cells

- Promotes the normal formation of red blood cells

Deficiencies:

- Neural tube defect: Spina Bifida

- Increased risk of heart disease, and stroke

- Anemia

- Red, sore tongue

- Diarrhea

- Cervical Cancer

Vitamin B12 (Cobalamin): The B12 vitamin is the most chemically complex of all the vitamins. It has been used as an antidote to cyanide poisoning. B12 plays a key role in the normal function of the brain and nervous system and the formation of blood. It is normally involved in metabolism of every cell of the body. This cannot be made by plants or animals. It can only be made by simple organisms, such as algae or bacteria, which have the enzymes required for its synthesis.

Functions:

- Help maintain nerve tissues

- Aids in reactions that build up protein and bone tissues

- Needed for normal red blood cell development with the help of the vitamin, folate

Deficiencies:

- Neurological disorders (nervousness, tingling sensations, brain degeneration)

- Pernicious anemia

- Fatigue

Vitamin C—Ascorbic Acid

Functions:

- Collagen formation: the protein of most connective tissues, skin and bone matrix

- Repairs wounds: forms scar tissue and helps healing

- Fights infections: enhances immune response

- Antioxidant: prevents damage from oxidation in cells. Stops action of free radicals that are formed by environmental factors or produced in the body during normal oxidation processes

- Helps with iron absorption

Deficiencies:

- Bleeding and bruising of weakened blood vessels, cartilage, tissues containing collagen

- Slow recovery from infections

- Poor wound healing

- Fatigue and depression

- Advanced stage is Scurvy, which has symptoms of swollen and bleeding gums

FIBER

Dietary fiber is an indigestible complex carbohydrate with limited nutritive value in itself but absorbs many times its weight in water and helps to move food through the digestive system more rapidly, aiding in the elimination of waste.

Dietary fiber also known as roughage or bulk includes all parts of plant foods that your body can't digest or absorb. Unlike other food components such as fats, proteins, or carbohydrates, which your body breaks down and absorbs, fiber isn't digested by your body. Therefore, it passes relatively intact through your stomach, small intestine, and colon and out of your body. It might seem like fiber doesn't do much, but it has several important roles in maintaining health.

Fiber is commonly classified into two categories: those that dissolve in water (soluble fiber) and those that do not dissolve in water (insoluble fiber).

Insoluble Fiber

This type of fiber promotes the movement of material through your digestive system and increases stool bulk, so it can be of benefit to those who struggle with constipation or irregular stools. Whole-wheat flour, wheat bran, nuts, and many vegetables are food sources of insoluble fiber.

Soluble Fiber

This type of fiber dissolves in water to form a gel-like material. It can help lower blood cholesterol and glucose levels. Soluble fiber is found in oats, peas, beans, apples, citrus fruits, carrots, barley, and psyllium.

Why We Need Fiber

Normalizes bowel movements: Dietary fiber increases the weight and size of your stool and softens it. A bulky stool is easier to pass, decreasing your chance of constipation. If you have loose, watery stools, fiber may also help to solidify the stool because it absorbs water and adds bulk to stool. For some, fiber may provide relief from Irritable Bowel Syndrome.

Helps maintain bowel integrity and health: A high fiber diet may lower your risk of developing hemorrhoids and small pouches in your colon (Diverticular disease). Some fiber is fermented in the colon. Researchers are looking at how this fermentation process may play a role in preventing diseases of the colon.

Lowers blood cholesterol levels: Soluble fiber found in beans, oats, flaxseed, and oat bran may help lower total blood cholesterol levels by lowering low-density lipoprotein (LDL) cholesterol or "bad" cholesterol levels. Epidemiologic studies have shown that increased fiber in the diet can reduce blood pressure and inflammation, which is also protective to heart health.

Helps control blood sugar levels: Fiber, particularly soluble fiber, can slow the absorption of sugar, which for people with diabetes can help improve blood sugar levels. A diet that includes insoluble fiber has been associated with a reduced risk of developing type 2 diabetes.

Aids in weight loss: High-fiber foods generally require more chewing time, which gives your body time to register that you are no longer hungry, making you less likely to overeat. Also, a high-fiber diet tends to make a meal feel larger and linger longer, so you stay full for a greater amount of time. High fiber diets also tend to be less "energy dense," which means they have fewer calories for the same volume of food.

Whole foods are generally a better source of fiber than fiber supplements. Refined or processed foods such as canned fruits and vegetables and pulp-free juice, white bread and pasta, and non-whole-grain cereals are lower in fiber content. The grain-refining process removes the outer coat (bran) from the grain, which lowers its fiber content. Similarly, removing the skin from fruits and vegetables decreases their fiber content.

High fiber foods are good for your health. However, adding too much fiber too quickly can promote intestinal gas, abdominal bloating, and cramping. By slowly adding fiber to your diet, you allow the natural bacteria in your digestive system to adjust to the change. Also drink plenty of water and *RyWhe* in order to make your stool soft and bulky.

Your best fiber choices:

- Grains and whole grain products

- Fruits

- Vegetables

- Beans, peas, and other legumes

- Nuts and seeds

CHOLESTEROL

Good vs. Bad

Cholesterol is a soft, waxy substance found among the lipids (fats) in the bloodstream and in all your body's cells. Surprise! Cholesterol itself is not bad. In fact, our body makes cholesterol in order for us to be healthy. It is an important part of a healthy body because it's used to form cell membranes. Cholesterol comes from two sources: our body and the food we eat. The liver and other cells in the body make 75 percent of the cholesterol in the bloodstream, whereas the other 25 percent comes from food consumption. Not only animal products have cholesterol. According to Dr. Lustig, fructose does more to increase bad cholesterol than fat or anything else we consume. He also states that since 1975, when fructose was introduced to our society, we have had an increase of bad cholesterol as well as high blood pressure and diabetes.

Why Do We Need Cholesterol?

Cholesterol is an essential structural component of cell membranes in mammals. It is also important for the manufacture of bile acids, steroid hormones, and vitamin D (vital for strong bones and teeth). Some examples of the steroid hormones include estrogen, testosterone, and cortisone. Cholesterol also aids in the transportation of fats around the body. This transportation is needed because fats do not dissolve in the body, so they must be carried from cell to cell. These transporters of fat are called lipoprotein. Lipoprotein means fat protein.

Components of Cholesterol

High-density lipoprotein and low-density lipoprotein, along with triglycerides and Lp(a) cholesterol, make up the total cholesterol count and can be determined through a blood test. The problem is not the cholesterol itself but the excessive levels of cholesterol in our bodies—particularly the bad LDL cholesterol, which contributes to plaque buildup in the arteries.

High-Density Lipoprotein (HDL) is known as the "good" cholesterol. HDL removes cholesterol from the blood. Higher levels of HDL are considered better for you. High HDL levels seem to protect against heart attack. Low levels of HDL can lead to increased risk of heart disease.

Low-Density Lipoprotein (LDL) is known as the "bad" cholesterol. LDL adds to plaque formation. When too much of this bad cholesterol, LDL, circulates in the blood, it can accumulate in the arteries that carry blood to the heart and brain. LDL, along with other components, can build up into plaque, which can clog the arteries; this is also known as atherosclerosis. Eating foods with saturated fat can lead to increased levels of LDL.

Triglycerides are a form of fat made in the body. People with high triglycerides often have a high total cholesterol level, including high LDL (bad) cholesterol and low HDL (good) cholesterol levels. Elevated triglycerides can be due to obesity/overweight, sedentary lifestyle, smoking, and a diet made up of more than 60 percent carbohydrates.

Lp(a) is a variation of LDL. At this time, Lp(a) is not widely understood, but it is thought to contribute to fatty deposits in arteries.

HDL+ LDL + Triglycerides + Lp(a) Cholesterol = *Total* cholesterol count

Cholesterol Levels

It is important to know what your cholesterol levels are and what they mean. When visiting your doctor, and he gives you your lipid panel results (cholesterol blood test), make sure you ask for HDL level and then the LDL level. If your HDL is high, don't panic and think that you need to be on unnecessary medication. The higher the HDL level is, the less LDL there is in the blood.

Total Cholesterol Levels

Less than 200 mg/dL:	Desirable level, lower risk of coronary heart disease
200-239 mg/dL:	Borderline High
240 and above:	High Cholesterol, twice as likely to have heart disease as someon

Below 40 (men) Below 50 (women)	Poor
50-59	Better
Above 60	Best

Less than 100	Optimal
100-129	Near optimal
130-159	Borderline high
160-189	High
Above 190	Very High

Less than 150	Normal
150-199	Borderline High
200-499	High
Above 500	Very High

Having total cholesterol levels lower than 200 lowers the risk of coronary heart disease. Individuals with total cholesterol levels of 240 or higher have twice the likelihood of developing heart disease than someone with less than 200.

HDL Levels:

Average HDL for men is 40-50

Average HDL for women is 50-60

LDL Levels:

Triglyceride Levels:

A triglyceride level of 150 mg/dl or higher is one of the risk factors for Metabolic Syndrome. Metabolic Syndrome increases the risk for heart disease and other disorders, including diabetes. People with high triglycerides often have a high total cholesterol level, including high LDL (bad) and low HDL (good).

Examples:

A female with a HDL of 55 or above and a LDL level of 100 for a total count of 155 is not high and should not be put on medication. Make sure you consult your physician.

A male with a HDL 45 or above with an LDL level of 100 for a total of 145 is not considered high. Consult your physician.

The problem is not the cholesterol itself but in the excessive cholesterol consumption—particularly the bad LDL cholesterol, which contributes to plaque buildup in the arteries. Make sure that you truly have high cholesterol before you begin any medications. Share your desires with your doctor before any mistakes are made. There are many who take unnecessary medications that can cause harm.

PROTEIN

Protein is a nutrient that the body needs to grow and maintain itself. Next to water, protein is the most plentiful substance in our bodies. Just about everyone knows that muscles are made of protein. Actually, every single cell in the body has some protein. In addition, other important parts of the body like hair, skin, eyes, and body organs are also made from protein. The composition of proteins in the body is like that muscle contains about 1/3 protein, bone about 1/5 part, and skin consists of 1/10 portion. The rest part of proteins is in the other body tissues and fluids. Even blood contains loads of proteins. In fact, the hemoglobin molecule, which carries blood through our body, is made entirely of proteins.

Protein is a source of nutrition for all the living organisms that are not able to produce or make energy through direct sunlight. It is the most important constituent of the body tissues, which are very useful in the growth and repair of cells. It is also very useful in supplying energy when carbohydrates and fats are not available. Some proteins have structural and mechanical roles in the body like they form struts and joints of cytoskeleton. Proteins are the primary substance of living organisms, as it provides the molecular machinery to the cells of living organisms.

Proteins are very important molecules in our cells. They are involved in virtually all cell functions. Each protein within the body has a specific function. Some proteins are involved in structural support while others are involved in bodily movement or defense against germs.

Proteins are made from simpler substances called amino acids. There are twenty amino acids in the protein that we eat every day. The body takes these amino acids and links them together in very long strings. This is how the body makes all of the different proteins it needs to function properly. Nine of the amino acids are called essential because our bodies cannot make them. These essential amino acids must come from the foods we eat. Proteins have distinct, three-dimensional shapes. Just as proteins vary in structure, they vary in function as well.

Proteins play a major role in ensuring your health and well being. There are innumerable functions of proteins in the body. The primary functions of proteins include building and repairing of body tissues, regulation of body processes, and formation of enzymes and hormones. Proteins aid in the formation of antibodies that enable the body to fight infection. Proteins serve as a major energy supplier. They also help in maintaining the water balance. Protein controls fluid volume and similarity in tissues throughout the body and blood.

This function contributes significantly to the water-balancing function. Proteins can maintain blood pH, as proteins are amphoteric and are able to cope with alkaline and acidic surroundings.

Signals are the communication between two cells. Proteins can carry signals because it has tendency to bind with other molecules, thus allowing the cells to pass information from one part of the body to others. This signaling allows the body to coordinate many cellular activities. Hormones and neurotransmitters, like insulin and serotonin respectively, are examples of proteins assisting in the controlling of body functions.

Protein Types

There are distinctive kinds of proteins, each performing a unique function in the body.

Antibodies are specialized proteins involved in defending the body from antigens (foreign invaders). One way antibodies destroy antigens is by immobilizing them so that they can be destroyed by white blood cells.

Contractile proteins are responsible for movement. Examples: actin and myosin. These proteins are involved in muscle contraction and movement.

Enzymes are proteins that facilitate biochemical reactions. They are often referred to as catalysts because they speed up chemical reactions. Examples include the enzymes lactase and pepsin. Lactase breaks down the sugar lactose found in milk. Pepsin is a digestive enzyme that works in the stomach to break down proteins in food.

Hormonal proteins are messenger proteins that help to coordinate certain bodily activities. Examples include insulin, oxytocin, and somatotropin. Insulin regulates glucose metabolism by controlling the blood-sugar concentration. Oxytocin stimulates contractions in females during childbirth. Somatotropin is a growth hormone that stimulates protein production in muscle cells.

Structural proteins are fibrous and stringy and provide support. Examples include keratin, collagen, and elastin. Keratins strengthen protective coverings, such as hair, quills, feathers, horns, and beaks. Collagen and elastin provide support for connective tissues, such as tendons and ligaments.

Storage proteins store amino acids. Examples include ovalbumin and casein. Ovalbumin is found in egg whites, and casein is a milk-based protein.

Transport proteins are carrier proteins that move molecules from one place to another in the body. Examples include hemoglobin and cytochromes. Hemoglobin transports oxygen through the blood. Cytochromes operate in the electron transport chain as electron carrier proteins.

Protein Consumption

Protein should account for 10 to 20 percent of the calories consumed each day. There are two types of proteins: complete (whole) protein and incomplete protein. Complete proteins are a source of protein that contain an adequate proportion of all nine essential amino acids. Eggs, milk, cheese, yogurt, and meats are sources of complete proteins. Incomplete proteins lack one or more of the essential amino acid. An incomplete protein can have all the essential amino acids but not in the correct proportions. Plant proteins are low in one or more essential amino acids.

Both plant and animal foods contain protein. Foods that provide all the essential amino acids are called high-quality proteins. Animal foods, like meat, fish poultry, eggs, and dairy products, are all high-quality protein sources. These are the foods people usually think of when they want to eat protein. The essential amino acids in animal products are in the right balance.

Foods that do not provide a good balance of all the essential amino acids are called lower quality proteins. Most fruits and vegetables are poor sources of protein. For vegetarians, vegans, and/or those who do not eat certain meats, fish, eggs, or dairy products, it is important to eat a variety of other foods in order to get enough protein in your diet. Protein plant foods contain lower-quality proteins.

People who do not eat animal products should add different types of plant foods together or within the same day to get the proper balance and amount of essential amino acids their bodies need. Combining beans and rice, or beans and corn, or peanut butter and bread will provide all of the essential amino acids in the right amounts. These food combinations mix foods from different plant groups to complement the amino acids provided by each. A small amount of animal product mixed with a larger amount of plant product can also meet a person's protein needs. By combining two of the following plant groups, you can make a higher-quality protein:

- Legumes: dry beans, peas, peanuts, lentils, and soybeans

- Grains: wheat, rye, rice, corn, and barley

- Seed nuts: sunflower seeds, pumpkin seeds, pecans, and walnuts

Protein Sources:

- Eggs

- Milk products: milk, cheese, and yogurt

- Meat: beef, poultry, fish lamb, and pork

- Whole grains

- Rice

- Corn

- Beans

- Legumes

- Oatmeal

- Peas

- Peanut butter

CARBOHYDRATES

Carbohydrates are the most important and readily available source of energy in our body. They contain the elements carbon, hydrogen, and oxygen. The first part of the name "carbo" means that they contain carbon. The second part of the name "hydr" means that they contain hydrogen. The last part of the name "ate" means that they have oxygen. In all carbohydrates, the ratio of hydrogen atoms to oxygen atoms is 2:1, just like water. According to the Dietary References published by the USDA, 45 percent to 65 percent of our energy should come from carbohydrates.

Carbohydrates play an important role in nutrition because they are a quick and efficient way to deliver energy to your cells. This energy can power your workouts and everyday activities. Carbohydrates are the body's main source of fuel and, as previously stated, are easily used by the body for energy. We obtain most of our carbohydrates in the form of "starch." Our digestive system turns starch into another carbohydrate called glucose. Glucose is carried around the body in the blood and is used by our tissues as a source of energy. Glucose in our food is absorbed without the need for digestion.

All tissues and cells in our body use glucose for energy. Carbohydrates are needed by the central nervous system, the kidneys, the brain, and muscles (including the heart) in order to function properly. Carbohydrates can be stored in the muscles and liver and later used for energy. One form of carbohydrates is important in intestinal health and waste elimination.

Carbohydrates are mainly found in starchy foods, like grain and potatoes, fruits, milk, and yogurt. Other foods like vegetables, beans, nuts, seeds, and cottage cheese contain carbohydrates but in lesser amounts.

Carbohydrates are one of the sixth classes and sources of nutrients that must be present in our daily diet in order to have good health and to control our weight. Carbohydrates are an essential structural component of living cells and a source of energy for animals. Carbohydrates include simple sugars with small molecules as well as macromolecular substances and are classified according to the number of monosaccharide group or sugars that they contain.

Carbohydrates come in a variety of forms, including sugars, starches, and fiber. Depending on their structure, they may also fall into one of the following two groups:

Simple carbohydrates include sugars like sucrose (table sugar), fructose (fruit sugar), and grape sugars, which are glucose or dextrose. Of all the simple sugars, glucose and dextrose are the simplest forms and more utilized by the body for energy since they are the most easily digested. Simple carbohydrates are not the recommend sources of carbohydrates. They cause spikes in blood sugar, which can facilitate fat storage and blunt fat burning. They also can cause you to feel tired later, once the original sugar high wears off.

Sugars added during food processing and refining have no nutrients and have many unhealthy side effects. If you do eat these simple sugars, make sure that you eat fiber with them. Fruits and vegetables naturally already have fiber.

Complex carbohydrates, on the other hand, contain three or more linked sugars, and thus require the body to work harder to break them down into glucose for energy. Some complex carbohydrates, like fruit fiber or vegetable fiber, for example, cannot be broken down by the body and are passed through undigested.

Complex carbohydrates speed up the metabolism because it takes more energy to digest them. Complex carbohydrates are considered the good carbohydrates because they are low in glycemic index. Therefore, complex carbohydrates do not cause quick spikes in blood sugar that simple, refined carbs would cause. These blood sugar spikes caused by refined carbs have been linked to increased risk for diabetes, metabolic syndrome, heart disease, and obesity.

Good sources of complex carbohydrates include whole grains like oatmeal, brown rice, and whole wheat, as well as fresh fruits and vegetables.

Fiber refers to certain types of carbohydrates that our body cannot digest. These carbohydrates pass through the intestinal tract intact and help to move waste out of the body. Diets that are low in fiber have been shown to cause problems such as constipation and hemorrhoids and increase the risk for certain types of cancers such as colon cancer. Diets high in fiber, however, have been shown to decrease risks for heart disease and obesity and help lower cholesterol. Foods high in fiber include fruits, vegetables, and whole grain products.

As fiber moves through the large intestine, bacteria break down much of the fiber. As they digest the fiber, these bacteria multiply and produce butyric acid, which has been shown to give protection against bowel cancer. Therefore, consuming fiber is important to intestinal health.

Some tips to increase fiber intake:

- Eat whole grain breads and brown rice

- Eat whole fruits rather than drink fruit juices

- Choose whole grain cereals at breakfast time

- Try raw vegetables for snacks rather than fatty or high-sugar snacks

- Keep the skins on fruits and vegetables (wash thoroughly)

For more information on Fiber, go to the "Fiber" chapter.

How Does the Body Process Carbohydrates and Sugar?

All carbohydrates are broken down into simple sugars. These sugars are absorbed into the bloodstream. As the sugar level rises, the pancreas releases a hormone called insulin, which is needed to move sugar from the blood into the cells where the sugar can be used as a source of energy.

Because complex carbohydrates digest slower than simple carbohydrates, they are less likely to convert into fat. Fruits are simple carbohydrates, however, because they are natural and raw with no added sugar, they have little effect on blood sugar. Complex carbohydrates must be part of your daily diet for a balanced diet. The carbohydrates in some foods, mostly those that contain simple sugars and highly refined grains, such as white flour and white rice, are easily broken down and cause your blood sugar level to rise quickly.

Starches are more complex, and the body has to break them down before they get into the blood stream. Complex carbohydrates (found in whole grains), on the other hand, are broken down more slowly, allowing blood sugar to rise more gradually, which your body converts to glucose for energy. Starches: (complex carbohydrates) found in foods such as starchy vegetables, grains, rice bread, bananas, barley, beans, brown rice, chickpeas, lentils, nuts oats, parsnips, potatoes, root vegetables, sweet corn, wholegrain cereals, whole grain breads, whole grain cereals, whole grain flour, whole grain pasta, and yams.

Refined vs. Unrefined

Grains come in two forms: refined and unrefined.

Refined grains have been stripped of their outer bran coating and inner germ during the milling process, leaving only the endosperm, resulting in the leftover grain having no nutrients whatsoever. They include white rice, white bread, and white pasta. Refined is the form that you want to stay away from as much as possible, especially if it is refined and then has high fructose corn syrup added (danger!). Refined with high fructose is a sure way to gain weight as well as to have a lot of health problems.

Unrefined or whole grain forms provide far more nutrients than their refined counterparts. In whole grains, the bran, germ, and endosperm are still present. The bran is an excellent source of fiber; the germ is a source of protein, vitamins, and minerals; and the endosperm supplies most of the carbohydrates, mainly in the form of starch. Whole grains are rich in phytochemicals and antioxidants, which help to protect against coronary heart disease, certain cancers, and diabetes. According to the USDA, individuals who eat more whole grain tend to have a healthier heart.

Most people get their whole grain from whole meal bread or whole grain breakfast cereals, such as porridge, muesli, or whole-wheat cereals. Choose a whole grain variety over processed or refined grains and look out for added sugar, high fructose corn syrup, salt, and any other additives. Look for the words *fructose* and *additives* of any kind and try to steer away from them.

Whole grains include wheat, oats, maize, barley, rye, millet, quinoa, and wild rice. *Whole wheat* means what it says; look for whole wheat on your labels.

Pasta

Pasta is made from dough of grain flour mixed with water. Most pasta is made from wheat; however, watch out for refined pasta. The nutritional quality of pasta, as well as its taste and texture, depends upon the flour used. Most pasta is also refined and processed. Macaroni means the pasta is made with semolina, farina, and/or flour made from refined durum wheat. Macaroni comes in many shapes: spaghetti, elbow macaroni, and shells. Also remember, the word semolina is an Italian word for "enriched white flour."

Pastas made with whole grain flours, such as whole pasta, are naturally the most nutrient-rich because the bran and germ of the grain have been left in. Most pasta is made with durum wheat, a hard wheat high in protein and gluten, which makes a dough that sticks together well and holds its shape. Remember when evaluating pasta: use the same criteria that you would use in comparing cereal: look for *whole grain*.

Egg noodles are made from flour, water, and egg (either egg white or whole eggs). At least 5.5 percent of the weight of the noodle must be from egg. Corn pasta has less protein than wheat pasta, but it is more easily digested by gluten-sensitive persons.

Carbohydrates are your body's main source of energy. They should be part of all meals, filling about a third of your plate. Although the amount of starches you eat should be regulated, you should never take them completely out of your diet. Remember, it is not the calories, it how the body processes or absorbs what you eat.

DIGESTION

Production of Digestive Juices

Digestion begins in the mouth with the saliva glands. Saliva enzymes digest the starch from food into smaller molecules. It is then pushed through the esophagus into the stomach. The second step occurs in the stomach lining. The lining produces stomach acid enzymes that digest proteins. Thirdly, the pancreas releases a juice that contains enzymes into the small intestine. This gastric juice contains a wide array of enzymes that break down carbohydrates, fats, and proteins in food. Also, the liver produces a bile juice. Bile is stored between meals in the gallbladder. The bile acid dissolves fat into the watery contents of the intestine, much like detergents that dissolve grease from a frying pan. After the fats are dissolved, it is digested by enzymes from the pancreas and from the lining of the intestine.

Absorption and
Transport of Nutrients

Most digested molecules of food, as well as water and minerals, are absorbed through the small intestine. Specialized cells allow absorbed materials to cross the mucosa into the blood, where they are carried off in the bloodstream to other parts of the body for storage or further chemical change. Mucosa is the membrane lining of bodily cavities and canals that lead to the outside, such as the digestive tract. This part of the process varies with different types of nutrients.

Carbohydrates: There are two main components of carbohydrates—crude fiber (i.e. mainly cellulose) and soluble sugars and starches. The digestible carbohydrates like sucrose and sugar are broken into simpler molecules by enzymes in the saliva and juice produced about the pancreas and in the lining of the small intestine. Starch is digested in two steps. First, enzymes in the saliva and pancreatic juice raise the sucrose into molecules called maltose. Then an enzyme in the lining of the small intestine split the maltose into glucose molecules that can be absorbed into the blood. Glucose is carried through the bloodstream to the liver where it is stored or used to provide energy for the work of the body.

Sugars are digested in one step. An enzyme in the lining of the small intestine digests sucrose, also known as table sugar, into glucose and fructose, which are absorbed through the intestine into the blood. Milk contains another type of sugar, lactose, which is changed into absorbable molecules by another enzyme in the intestinal lining. Fiber is indigestible and moves through the digestive tract without being broken down by enzymes. Many foods contain both soluble and insoluble fiber. Soluble fiber dissolves easily in water and takes on a soft, gel-like texture in the intestines. Insoluble fiber, on the other hand, passes essentially unchanged through the intestines.

Proteins: Proteins are foods such as meat, eggs, and beans consisting of giant molecules of proteins that must be digested by enzymes before they can be used to build and repair body tissues. An enzyme in the juice of the stomach starts the digestion of the swallowed protein. Once in the small intestine, several enzymes from pancreatic juice and from lining of the intestine complete the breakdown of the huge protein molecules into small molecules called amino acids. These small molecules can be absorbed through small intestine into the blood and then be carried to all parts of the body to build the cell membranes and other parts of cell.

Fats: Fat molecules are a rich source of energy for the body. The first step in digestion of a fat, such as butter, is to dissolve it into the watery content of the intestine. The bile acids produced by the liver dissolve fat into tiny droplets and allow pancreatic and intestinal enzymes to break the large fat molecules into smaller ones called fatty acids and cholesterol. The bile acids combine with the fatty acids and cholesterol and help these molecules move into the cells of the mucosa. In these cells, the small molecules are formed back into large ones, most of which pass into vessels called lymphatic vessels near the intestine. These small vessels carry the reformed fat to the veins of the chest, and the blood carries the fat storage depots in different parts of the body.

Vitamins: Another vital part of food that is absorbed through the small intestines is vitamins. The two types of vitamins are classified by the fluid in which they can be dissolved: water-soluble vitamins (all of the B vitamins and vitamin C) and fat-soluble vitamins (vitamins A, D, E, and K). Fat-soluble vitamins are stored in the liver and fatty tissue of the body, whereas water-soluble vitamins are not easily stored, and excess amounts are flushed out in the urine.

Water and salt: Most of the material absorbed through the small intestine is water in which salt is dissolved. The salt and water come from the food and liquid you ingest and the juices secreted by many digestive glands.

Digestion Regulators

The digestive process is controlled by hormone regulators. The major hormones that control the functions of the digestive system are produced and released by cells in the mucosa of the stomach and small intestine. These hormones are released into the blood of the digestive tract, travel back to the heart and through the arteries, and return to the digestive system where they stimulate digestive juices and cause organ movement. The main hormones that control digestion are gastrin, secretin, and cholecystokinin (CCK).

Gastrin causes the stomach to produce an acid for dissolving and digesting some foods. Gastrin is also necessary for normal cell growth in the lining of the stomach, small intestine, and colon.

Secretin causes the pancreas to send out a digestive juice that is rich in bicarbonate. The bicarbonate helps neutralize the acidic stomach contents as they enter the small intestine. Secretin also stimulates the stomach to produce pepsin, an enzyme that digests protein and stimulates the liver to produce bile.

CCK causes the pancreas to produce the enzymes of pancreatic juice and causes the gallbladder to empty. It also promotes normal cell growth of pancreas.

Additional hormones in the digestive system that regulate appetite are ghrelin and peptide YY. Ghrelin and peptide are important hormones because they work on the brain to help regulate the intake of food for energy.

Ghrelin is produced in the stomach and upper intestine in the absence of food in the digestive system and stimulates appetite.

Peptide YY is produced in the digestive tract in response to a meal in the system and inhibits appetite.

SYNTHETIC VS. NATURAL

Five years ago I was taking as many synthetic vitamins as I could possibly take. I now know that the very thing that I thought was good for me was making me sick. The fat-soluble vitamins A, D, E, and K were not even being processed or absorbed in my body. In fact, they were becoming toxins in my body, causing sickness and disease. These synthetic vitamins and minerals were toxic themselves. When I found out the process of how synthetic vitamins were made, I became sick to my stomach.

Natural

Whole food ingredients are naturally and easily absorbed by the body. They are made from pure, raw materials that contain hundreds of cofactors, other nutrients that the body needs to absorb vitamins, while synthetic ingredients do not. These micronutrients are indispensable for proper vitamin absorption and maximum utilization. When cofactors are missing, as they are in synthetic vitamins, the body may treat the vitamin as a foreign substance and eliminate it or pass it whole. Natural foods solve these problems while providing vitamins the body can absorb. Natural vitamins and minerals from the food you eat will not become toxic; however, if you take synthetic vitamins and minerals, you can become toxic, and more than likely, you will.

When we say *natural* or *whole* food, we're speaking of products that contain a total family of micronutrients, known and unknown, just as they are found in nature. For instance, in nature, beta-carotene is part of a family of carotenoids. It is never found alone. Carrots and tomatoes have alpha-carotene, beta-carotene, cantozantheen, gamma-carotene, omega-carotene, etc. And although beta-carotene is a great antioxidant, cantozantheen is already known to be an even more effective antioxidant. In other words, by isolating beta-carotene from its family of carotenoids, the experts have taken away an even more beneficial antioxidant.

In short, whole vitamins are made from food and are live replacement parts for your body, while synthetic vitamins are dead and comprised of laboratory-derived chemical reactions.

Synthetic

Did you know that most vitamins on the market claiming to be natural only have to be 10 percent natural to make this claim? Many "natural" vitamins have synthetics added to increase potency or to standardize the amount in a capsule or batch. In addition, a salt form is added to increase stability of the nutrient (i.e. acetate, bitartrate, chloride, gluconate, hydrochloride, nitrate, succinate). Most of the food supplements sold on the market today are synthetic. The biological activity is reduced by 50 percent and sometimes even to 70 percent in synthetic form.

What you should know is that if you are taking synthetic vitamins or minerals, they are not doing you any good, and your body will not process them. The water-soluble vitamins will just pass through you via urine, with no benefits. The fat-soluble vitamins, however, will become toxins in your body; they have no way of being absorbed because the body will not recognize them.

Synthetic means that a chemist attempted to reconstruct the exact structure of the crystalline molecule by chemically combining molecules from other sources. These sources are not living foods but dead chemicals. Crystalline means that natural food has been treated with various chemicals, solvents, heat, and distillations to reduce it down to one specific, pure, crystalline vitamin. In this process, all the synergists, which are term impurities, are destroyed. There is no longer anything natural in the action of crystalline vitamins.

Most synthetically produced vitamins and supplements are chemical compounds that cannot be found in nature; hence the human body does not recognize these ingredients, which can result in unanticipated reactions. The body knows the difference between real and fake, and it always prefers real. Dr. Charles Schneider, PhD, professor of Chemistry, University of Cincinnati, states that, in a laboratory, chemists can duplicate seawater that is chemically identical to natural seawater, but if you put fish in this synthetic water, they will die. Obviously, there is a life-supporting difference between natural and synthetic.

There are many negative health and environmental impacts from synthetic ingredients in vitamins and supplements. Get this! Many synthetics are made from coal tar derivatives, the same substances that cause throat cancer for tobacco smokers, and no cofactors are present. Surely your body can tell the difference between food and coal tar.

Some people are allergic to the chemicals used as a base for synthetic vitamins. Some are toxic, including nicotine, coal tars, and alloxal. Medical findings indicate that synthetic substances may cause reactions in chemically susceptible individuals. Interestingly, the same individuals can tolerate naturally derived vitamins.

The fat-soluble vitamins include vitamins A, D, E, and K. Because they are soluble in fat (lipids), these vitamins tend to build up in the body's fat tissues, fat deposits, and liver. The storage capability makes the fat-soluble vitamins potentially toxic when consumed in high doses. Harm comes in when the synthetic versions of these vitamins are consumed rather than food-based vitamins that the body knows how to metabolize.

Dr. Schneider uses the image in a mirror to help relate synthetic vitamins. It looks like the real thing but doesn't function like the real thing. Which would you rather have? The food in the mirror or the real food? I say to my fellow women, do you want a diamond or a cubic zirconia (fake)? Fake is not real; that is why it is called fake or a copy. Which has the most value?

Natural versus synthetic is simple. It's real versus fake. You do the math; which has the most value: a diamond or a cubic zirconia?

SEVEN ELIMINATION SYSTEMS

I believe that God purposely and uniquely designed the body to heal itself naturally. He gave the human body seven elimination systems that will remove toxins and all waste from the body. These systems are God's way of keeping the body healthy. As long as we eat a balanced diet and do a little exercise, we will have quality life—a life that is full of vitality and medication free. We can have a sound body and mind with health and longevity. The only reason to go to the doctor's office would be for a yearly wellness check.

The seven elimination systems are:

1. Liver

2. Lungs

3. Kidneys

4. Lymphatic System

5. Colon

6. Blood

7. Skin

We should not suppress these systems. The seven elimination systems are the way for the body to remove toxins from the body on its own with any help from man. They are God's way of the body healing itself. However, we are always suppressing these systems. We are constantly changing what is natural by using chemicals and poisons to suppress what needs to work naturally.

Liver

Your liver is one of the largest and most important organs in your body. The liver is the body's main factory. It metabolizes food, filters toxins, and converts ingredients into substances that are needed in all parts of the body. When healthy, the liver will store vitamins, sugars, fats, and other nutrients from the food that you eat. The liver builds chemicals that your body needs to stay healthy and breaks down harmful substances, like alcohol and other toxic (poisonous) chemicals. It also removes waste products from your blood and makes sure that your body has just the right amount of other chemicals that it needs.

The liver is a metabolically active organ responsible for many vital life functions. However, the primary functions are:

- Bile production and excretion

- Excretion of bilirubin, cholesterol, hormones, and drugs

- Metabolism of fats, proteins, and carbohydrates

- Enzymes activation

- Storage of glycogen, vitamins, and minerals

- Synthesis of plasma proteins, such as albumin and clotting factors

- Blood detoxification and purification

The liver contains many enzymes. Some of these enzymes in the liver are used for toxin processing. Blood flows through the liver where toxins in the blood can be processed. Some of the enzymes work to inactivate toxins to keep them from damaging the body. Enzymes can also break down compounds in the blood or modify them so that they stay dissolved and can then be excreted via the kidneys or other methods.

Lungs

Your lungs are in charge of breathing, so you better take care of them. The best way to care for the lungs is to give them plenty of exercise. Deep breathing of fresh air is the best exercise. Another way to keep your lungs healthy is to not smoke. Smoking is not good for any part of your body, especially your lungs. Also be careful of cleaning chemicals, as they are equally toxic to the lungs.

One toxin that can rapidly build up if not constantly eliminated is carbon dioxide. This toxin is created through normal metabolic processes throughout the body and is collected by the blood. Oxygen-rich blood is transported from the heart to the tissues through the blood vessels. Once it reaches the capillaries, the blood releases its oxygen and picks up carbon dioxide. The blood then transports carbon dioxide back to the lungs, releasing it into the air through process of breathing. According to the National Heart Lung and Blood institute, sensors in the brain and blood vessels monitor the level of carbon dioxide and adjust the breathing rate to ensure that it does not build up and damage the body.

Kidneys

The kidneys regulate the body's fluid volume, mineral composition, and acidity by excreting and reabsorbing water and inorganic electrolytes. This helps balance substances, which include sodium, potassium, chloride, calcium, magnesium, sulfate, phosphate, and hydrogen in the body and keep their normal concentration in the extracellular fluid. The body fluid volume, which is regulated by the kidneys, is related to blood volume and the blood pressure in your arteries.

The basic function of the kidneys is to filter waste products out of the blood, concentrate them into urine, and then eliminate that urine. Filtration actually occurs within a small kidney structure called the nephron. Each kidney has about 1 million nephrons. Inside the nephron, tiny blood vessels release the waste products they are carrying, which are picked up by a collecting tube. According to the national kidney and urological disease information clearinghouse, a complicated chemical balance within the nephron allows only the waste products to be removed into the urine-collecting tube. Urine is then passed from the kidney to the bladder and then excreted.

Lymphatic System

The lymphatic is the body's filter system, which supports immune function. A healthy lymphatic system filters out bacteria and other foreign particles. The lymphatic system is often referred to as the immune system. It is also considered part of the cardiovascular system. Regular exercise is the best treatment that your lymphatic system can receive.

Excess fluid that leaks out of capillaries to bathe the body's cells is collected by the vessels of the lymphatic system and returned to the blood. By doing so, the lymphatic system maintains the fluid balance in the body. The lymphatic system further assists the cardiovascular system in absorbing nutrients from the small intestine.

These necessary actions, however, are only part of the system's vitally important overall function. It is the body's main line of defense against foreign invaders such as bacteria and viruses. The lymphatic system is responsible for body immunity, filtering harmful substances out of tissue fluid (which fills the spaces between the cells) before that fluid is returned to the blood and the rest of the body. A natural herb by the name of arabinogalactan is a natural cleanser to the lymphatic system. Arabinogalactan comes from the wood of the larch tree and is approved by the FDA as a dietary fiber. Larch trees are common to New England, the upper Midwest, and much of Canada.

Colon

The colon is part of the digestive system, which is a series of bodily organs beginning at the mouth and ending with the anus. The colon is responsible for the final stages of the digestive process. The colon's function is threefold: to absorb the remaining water and electrolytes from indigestible food matter, to accept and store food remains that were not digested in the small intestine, and to eliminate solid waste (feces) from the body.

The colon works to maintain the body's balance. It absorbs certain vitamins, processes indigestible material (such as fiber), and stores waste before it is eliminated. Within the colon, the mixture of fiber, small amounts of water, and vitamins, etc. mix with mucus and the bacteria that live in the large intestine, beginning the formation of feces.

The colon absorbs vitamins, salts, nutrients, and water. When these essential, life-giving ingredients are being properly absorbed, we feel good. But when the colon is not working well, it begins to absorb toxins into the blood stream rather than expel them. The result is a myriad of problems, ranging from constipation and gas to candida, diverticulitis, and other various chronic health issues.

The colon hosts many bacteria. Over one hundred trillion microorganisms (bacteria) call the colon home. There are more microorganisms in the colon than there are human cells contained within the skin, heart, bone, brain, and the rest of the body combined. A proper balance of healthy bacteria must be maintained inside the colon to avoid being constantly plagued with ailments.

Bowels movements are basic for your health. If you don't have a least one bowel movement per day, you are already walking your way toward disease. All the refined sugar, white flour, and the hormone and anti-biotic-filled meats we constantly ingest constitute an assault on our bodies.

Begin a diet rich in raw fruits and vegetables with very little or no processed and refined foods at all. Hydration of the digestive system will improve colon health. Drinking an equivalent number of ounces of water to your body weight every day can do this. Also hydrating the colon through colon hydrotherapy has proven to be very beneficial to re-establishing health.

Blood

The blood is a liquid organ that transfers and transports substances throughout the body. It is what delivers the needed substances like nutrients and oxygen to those areas that are in need. Blood also transports carbon dioxide and other waste products away from the cells to the lungs, kidneys, and digestive system. From these organs, the waste is removed from the body. In addition, the blood also helps fight infection in open cuts in the body.

Whole blood contains three types of blood cells: red blood cells, white blood cells, and platelets. Red blood cells, also called RBCs or erythrocytes, contain iron-rich protein called hemoglobin, giving blood its characteristic red color. White blood cells, also called

WBCs or leukocytes, help fight diseases. Platelets, or thrombocytes, help in blood clotting. These cells that make up the whole blood travel through the circulatory system suspended in a yellowish fluid called plasma. Plasma is 90 percent water and contains nutrients, proteins, hormones, and waste products. Whole blood is a mixture of blood cells and plasma. Red clover and chlorella are wonderful natural cleansers of the blood system. A regular excise routine stimulates the blood system and assists the body in eliminating waste.

Skin

The skin is the body's largest organ. By sweating naturally, you assist in cleansing the skin and keeping it elastic and healthy. Going to a sauna and sweating is a wonderful health regimen for the skin. The skin functions in homeostasis include protection of body temperature, sensory reception, water balance, synthesis of vitamins and hormones, and absorption of materials.

The skin's primary functions are to serve as a barrier to the entry of microbes and viruses and to prevent water and extracellular fluid loss. Acidic secretions from skin glands also retard the growth of fungi. Melanocytes form a second barrier: protection from the damaging effects of ultraviolet radiation. When a microbe penetrates the skin (or when the skin is breached by a cut) the inflammatory response occurs. Functions of the skin include protection against:

- Mechanical impact such as pressure and stroke

- Thermic impact such as heat or cold

- Environmental impact such as chemicals, the sun's UV radiation

- Bacteria

Intoxicating Our Bodies

Now that you know the elimination systems, let us discuss how you are probably ruining them. Daily, our bodies are trying to expel or discharge waste and/or toxins. And we must let it expel if we don't want to have a diseased, sick body. Let nature run its course. If your nose is running, blow it, then drink plenty of water and the natural drink RyWhe. Let whatever waste and toxins that are in your body move out naturally.

Women, you should be concerned with how you are managing your menstrual cycle. You should never take medications to stop your cycle. The body uses menstruation to eliminate toxins. Therefore, it acts as a natural, monthly cleansing. The hormones in women's bodies help to keep bones body strong and skin soft and resilient. If this is a way of the body cleaning itself, monthly removing toxins, why would you not let it remove toxins? I believe that this is one of the reason women have breast cancer as well as other feminine problems.

Another way in which toxins can be eliminated from the body is through sweat. Some toxins and waste products in the blood are able to diffuse into the sweat glands. As a result, when the body excretes sweat, some toxins are excreted as well. Sweating is normally not able to process nearly as many toxins as urine production by the kidneys, but it provides an auxiliary method of toxin elimination. Yet we want to stop this process as well!

Women do not want to sweat. According to the International Hyperhidrosis Society, women are taking injections and using antiperspirant deodorant (if it is "anti," then it is not good) to stop sweating. Botox injections can help relieve excess sweating when botulinum (a toxin that can cause paralysis) is injected into the underarms. The toxin then influences the chemical that activates the sweats glands, causing the glands not to be activated. Sweat is the body's natural way of cooling itself along with other healthy things. We are taking these toxins and chemicals and putting them under our arms, giving them direct access to our lymphatic systems. I strongly believe this is the reason that there is so much sickness and early death for women.

Think about what you are doing to yourself. Eat a healthy and balanced diet. Look and feel good naturally. You can look and feel younger just by taking care of yourself and avoid things that are dangerous and may not be necessary to put in or on your body.

THE HIERARCHY OF LIFE'S NEEDS

In life there is a hierarchy of needs—biologically, physically, and mentally. Mentally the hierarchy of your psyche is explained in Maslow's Hierarchy of Needs pyramid. In the physical aspect, the USDA developed a food pyramid that lists the amount of each food group we should eat. After much studying and introspection, I have developed two pyramids for the biological realm of life. My pyramids of Nutrition and Nutrients go to the very root of life.

The relationship between these charts—the Maslow, the USDA, and the Smith's Hierarchy of Nutrition and Nutrients Charts—are all in one accord. The foundation of each pyramid must be solid in order to move to the next level. Each chart expresses a basic level from which the rest stems from. Also each chart addresses the fundamental needs for life. The absence of one can lead to a "Failure to Thrive" state or lead to a dysfunctional state of being.

Maslow Hierarchy of Needs

According to Maslow, there are five general types of needs: biological/physiological, security/safety, belonging/love, esteem, and self-actualization.

Physiological needs are those required to sustain life, such as air, water, food, sleep, sex, and excretion. If you are hungry, your motivation is to get food, and you will not move to another level until the hunger is satisfied.

Safety needs include living in a safe area, medical insurance, job security, and financial reserves. Once physiological needs are met, one's attention turns to safety and security in order to be free from the threat of physical and emotional harm.

Love and/or *belonging* is a social need. Once a person has met the lower level physiological and safety needs, higher level motivators awaken. The first level of higher level need is social needs. Social needs are those related to interaction with others and may include friendship, belonging to a group, and giving and receiving love.

Esteem needs follow after a person feels that they "belong." The urge to attain a degree of importance emerges. Esteem needs can be categorized as external motivators and internal motivators. Internally motivating esteem needs are those such as self-esteem, accomplishment, and self-respect. External esteem needs are those such as reputation, recognition, and attention.

Self-actualization is the highest level of need. People who reach self-actualization tend to have motivators such as truth, justice, wisdom, and meaning.

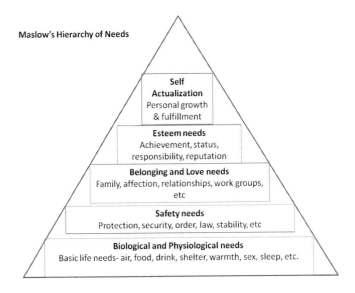

Maslow's Hierarchy of Needs

Self Actualization
Personal growth & fulfillment

Esteem needs
Achievement, status, responsibility, reputation

Belonging and Love needs
Family, affection, relationships, work groups, etc

Safety needs
Protection, security, order, law, stability, etc

Biological and Physiological needs
Basic life needs- air, food, drink, shelter, warmth, sex, sleep, etc.

The Maslow's Hierarchy of Needs chart explains that we must satisfy each need in succession, starting with the first, which deals with the most obvious needs for survival itself. Only when the lower levels are satisfied can we be concerned with the higher level needs, which include influence and personal development. Human needs arrange themselves in hierarchies of pre-potency. That is to say, the appearance of one need usually rests on the prior satisfaction of another, more pre-potent need.

Man is a perpetually wanting animal. Also, no need or drive can be treated as if it were isolated or discrete; every drive is related to the state of satisfaction or dissatisfaction of other drives. For instance, a person that lacks esteem or love may manifest this lack with a dissatisfaction with food. This leads to the eating disorders of anorexia, bulimia, and compulsive overeating.

Correlating with the Hierarchy of Needs pyramid is Maslow's Motivation Theory. The basis of his Motivation Theory is that human beings are motivated by unsatisfied needs and that certain lower factors must be satisfied before trying to acquire items at a higher level. Take a child that does not feel safe at home or have food to eat. When he gets to school, he will not be focused on learning or socializing with other students, as his basic needs of food and security are not met. We are trying to move this child to the next level when he has not mastered the first one. Please note that motivation theory is not synonymous with behavior theory, the motivations are only one class of determinants for behavior. While behavior is almost always motivated, it is almost always biologically, culturally, and situationally determined as well.

There are two groups among Maslow's Needs: deficiency needs (D-needs) and being needs (B-needs).

Deficiency needs are those needs that arise due to a deprivation: physiological, safety, love, and esteem. With the exception of the most fundamental need, physiological, if these "deficiency needs" are not met, the body gives no physical indication, but deficiency will manifest itself in other ways. The individual may feel anxious or tense.

Being needs are not from a lack of something but rather from a desire to grow as a person: self-actualization. Self-actualized persons have frequent occurrences of peak experiences, which are energized moments of profound happiness and harmony. According to Maslow, only a small percentage of the population reaches the level of self-actualization.

Maslow also coined the term "Metamotivation" to describe the motivation of people who go beyond the scope of the basic needs and strive for constant betterment. Metamotivated people are driven by B-needs (being needs), instead of deficiency needs (D-Needs). Each level of D-needs must be satisfied before a person can act unselfishly or reach a level of self-actualization. Conversely, if the things that satisfy our lower order needs are swept away, we are no longer concerned about the maintenance of our higher order needs. Satisfying needs is healthy, while preventing gratification makes us sick or act evil.

USDA Food Pyramid

The USDA Food Pyramid is a chart developed by the US government to educate its citizens on the daily dietary requirements. I consider this chart to be of the physical aspect of life. Recently they have rearranged their food pyramid, yet I have used the older version to create the Nutrition Nutrient Chart.

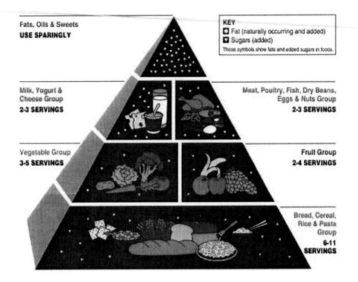

Source: http://www.cnpp.usda.gov/Publications/
MyPyramid/OriginalFoodGuidePyramids/FGP/
FGPPamphlet.pdf

The Smith's Hierarchy of Nutrition and Nutrients

Biologically, it all begins with the foods we eat. Life begins with the food that you eat. You are not only what you eat; you are also how your body digests or absorbs what you eat. I am truly amazed at how food affects the very basis of life. Just as there is no life without food, there is no life with the wrong foods. So that being said, food is the force of life. Without it there is no life, and with the wrong food, there is no life.

The lack of nutrition results in system breakdowns, sickness, diseases, and even death. When you eat the wrong foods, eliminate whole food groups according to a fad diet, or starve yourself, you are severely slowing down your metabolism and draining your enzyme bank. I have previously stated that once you have depleted your enzymes, there is no life. Enzymes are so vital for life. Remember you are born with metabolic enzymes and digestive enzymes, and unless you get the food enzymes to help these enzymes, you will become sick and, yes, maybe even have an early death.

It has been suggested that the respiratory system and the digestive system are the only two ways in which we become sick. If the food and drinks we consume, nutrition and nutrients, drastically affects one of the only two ways we can become sick, then we must also know that nutrition and nutrients are central to our well being.

Life's foundation begins with enzymes. Enzymes are the catalyst for all living cells, therefore, life. They are the force of life. They are involved in all functions of the body from brain processes and basic movement to organ function. We feel, hear, and see all due to enzymatic processes. Enzymes breakdown fats and improve aging skin.

Smith's Hierarchy of Nutrients

The Smith's Hierarchy of Nutrients chart is built from the foundation of the Maslow and the USDA charts. The Smith's chart is complementary to the other charts. It shows the existence of life and the importance of the

parallel of these charts of life. The grave difference of
the Smith's chart is the very essence of life. Our most
basic needs are innate. The nutrient goes to the core of
life—enzymes. Without enzymes, there is no life, as
vitamins, minerals, or hormones cannot do any work
without enzymes.

The Maslow Hierarchy of Needs states that we
must satisfy each need in turn, starting with the first,
which deals with the most obvious needs for survival.
Therefore, I begin with enzymes because, without them,
nothing else matters; every living thing has enzymes,
even plants. We are born with trillions of enzymes that
help keep our bodies existing, and once these enzymes
are used up, life is no more.

Level I: Enzymes

Our bodies contain trillions of enzymes that continually renew, maintain, and protect us; no person plant
or animal could exist without enzymes. Without them,
there would be no breathing, no digestion, no growth,
no blood coagulation, no perception of the senses, and
no reproduction.

Level II: Probiotics

It has been estimated that there are more microbial
cells existing in the body than human cells. Probiotic
liberally means, "life giving." Probiotics repopulate the
good bacteria that can help kill the bad bacteria and
fight infection. Gut flora, intestinal flora, microflora,
and direct-fed microorganisms (DFM) probiotics help
maintain the natural balance of organisms (microflora)

in the intestines. They are living, microscopic organisms such as bacteria, viruses, and yeasts that play a vital role in the fermentation and digestion of carbohydrates and aid in the digestion of fats and proteins. They prevent bloating, gas, and yeast overgrowth.

Level III: Amino Acids

Amino acids have a stimulant effect needed for muscle metabolism and tissue repair, helps with sexual arousal, may help with indigestion due to lack of stomach acid, aids in removing heaving metals from the system, helps prevent fertility problems, improves concentration, helps lower high serum triglycerides.

Examples: histidine, leucine, isoleucine, lysine, methione, phenylalnine, theonine, tryptophan, valine

The SMITH'S HEIRARCHY of NUTRIENTS
©

Healthy Mind Healthy Body   *Healthy Body Healthy Mind*

Level V

PHYTONUTRIENTS

Anti-bacterial, anti-fungal, anti-viral, anti-carcinogenic, lowers the risk of stomach and colon cancer. bind toxic materials and escort them out of the body. Helps build healthy blood, protect against cancer and a powerful wound healer. Blocks the uptake of cholesterol and excrete it from the body thus help in to prevent heart disease also halts the development of tumors in breast colon and prostate glands, anti-inflammatory, stop cancer cell formation.

Level IV

ANTIOXIDANTS

Protects our cells from free radicals, Compounds that protect against cell damage, Plays a role in preventing the development of chronic diseases as cancer, heart disease, stroke, Alzheimer's, Rheumatoid arthritis and cataracts, keeps the elasticity of capillary wall.

Level III

AMINO ACIDS

Building blocks of protein, important that one maintains a steady and balanced supply of these nutrients proper body, performance, muscles building and repair, Sexual arousal, may help with nerve deafness

Level II

PROBIOTICS

Healthy bacteria, living microorganism, maintains the natural balance of organisms (microflora) in the intestines. Live microscopic living organisms, such as bacteria, and yeasts have a vital role in the fermentation and digestion of carbohydrates and aid in the digesting fats and proteins, important for bowel function, prevention of colon cancer, can lower cholesterol, reduces inflammation, help with mineral absorption

Level I

ENZYMES/ALKALINE

Enzymes are the catalyst for all living cells (LIFE). It is the catalyst for life force. Is involved in all functions of the body, basic movement, to the function of our organs, thoughts that come from our brain move, feel, hear, see, enhance blood, breaks down fats, helps to shed excess weight, enhance mental capacity, improves aging skin

Level IV: Antioxidants

Antioxidants block the process of oxidation by neutralizing free radicals. In doing so, the antioxidants themselves become oxidized. Antioxidants are substance of nutrients in our foods that can prevent or slow the oxidative damage to our body. Antioxidants act as free radical scavengers and hence prevent and repair damage done by free radicals.

Examples: beta carotene (pre-cursor of vitamin A) , vitamins A, C, E, and the minerals selenium, zinc, and magnesium.

Level V: Phytonutrients

Phytonutrients (also referred to as phytochemicals) are compounds found in plants. They serve various functions in plants, helping to protect the plant's vitality. Phytonutrients are essential for optimum health and longevity. These chemicals, found in minute amounts in plant foods, provide thousands of reasons: to protect itself against bacteria, viruses, and fungi; to sustain its life functions such as photosynthesis; and to acts as antioxidants. Researchers are still discovering the ways in which phytochemicals may protect against certain diseases, boost immune system responses, and mediate enzymes functions and hormonal actions.

Smith's Hierarchy
of Nutrition

Level I: Carbohydrates

Carbohydrates are the most important sources of energy for the human body. Carbohydrate is a compound containing carbon, hydrogen, and oxygen atoms. Most are known as grain sugars, starches, and fibers. Carbohydrates are also level I on the USDA food pyramid.

The two bottom layers of the USDA food pyramid (breads and grains, fruits, and vegetables) consist of foods high in carbohydrates; sugar is also a carbohydrate (as honey, molasses, syrup, and other sweeteners). Carbohydrate is the food that most influences blood glucose levels. So tracking the amount of carbohydrates in your diet is one way to plan meals.

Carbohydrates are key to your diet. Do not eliminate them; learn how to use them for your best result. Make them work for you, not you work for them.

Level II: Proteins

Protein helps your body to build and retain muscle. Proteins can also be used for fuel. It also takes double the time to change protein into smaller molecules. Proteins play a major role in ensuring your health and well-being. There are innumerable functions of protein in the body. However, the primary functions of proteins include building and repairing of body tissues, regulation of body processes, and formation of enzymes and hormones. Proteins aid in the formation of antibodies that enable the body to fight infection. Proteins serve as a major energy supplier. There are distinctive kinds of proteins, each performing a unique function in the body. Proteins form a major part of your body, next to water.

The composition of proteins in the body is like that muscle contains about 1/3 protein, bone contains about 1/5 protein, skin consist about 1/10. The other parts of the body tissues, fluids, and the blood contain large amounts of protein. Also, the hemoglobin is made of molecule from proteins.

Proteins form an important nutrient component of the body. Made up of essential and non-essential amino acids, it helps in building and repairing muscles and bones and restoring body cells.

Protein-rich foods are those such as beans, nuts, poultry, fish, and eggs.

Level III: Fats/Lipids

Another supply of energy comes from fats. Fat makes up 70 percent of the brain and the nerves that run every system in the body. So it stands to reason that the better the fat in the diet, the better the brain (the good fat). The average America brain is getting fat, but it's not getting the right kind of fat.

Your brain is the master gland that sends chemical messengers throughout the body. It tells each organ how to work. An important group of these chemical messengers are the prostaglandins (called this because they were originally discovered in the prostate gland). Prostaglandins initiate the body's self-repair system.

When the cells of the human body and the human brain are deprived of the essential fatty acids they need to grow and function, the cells will try to build replacement fatty acids that are similar but may actually be harmful. High blood levels of "replacement fatty acids" are associated with diets that are high in hydrogenated fats and diets that contain excessive amounts of omega-6 fatty acids. Levels of replacement fatty acids have been found to be elevated in persons suffering from depression or attention deficit disorder. A diet rich in omega-3 fatty acids (such as the LNA from flax oil or the EPA from fish oils) not only provides the body with healthy fats, but it also lowers the blood level of potentially harmful ones, such as cholesterol and possibly even reversing the effects of excess trans fatty acids. The retina of the eye contains a high concentration of the fatty acid DHA, which the body forms from nutritious fats in the diet. The more nutritious the fat, the better the eye can function. And since most people are visual learners, better eyes mean better brains. This is where you can see the necessity for vitamin A, the fat-soluble vitamin; it is only absorbed in fat.

Fat helps food to stay in the stomach longer, giving a greater sense of satisfaction and preventing hunger soon after meals. Fat also helps the body produce endorphins (natural substances) in the brain that produce pleasurable feelings. Diets too low in fat (9 less 25 percent) may trigger cravings.

Levels IV: Vitamins

Vitamins are chemical compounds necessary for normal growth, maintenance of health, and reproduction. There are thirteen vitamins currently identified as essential for maintaining good health; the body cannot survive without them. Vitamins are elements for the human body that contained within food substances. They help the body use energy, maintain normal body tissue, act as a regulator, and are only needed in small amounts.

Of the thirteen needed vitamins, four can be produced in the body. Biotin, pantothenic, acid, and vitamin K are made in the human intestine and usually in adequate amounts to meet the body's needs. Sunlight on the skin surfaces can produce sufficient amounts of vitamin D. The remaining vitamins must be supplied in the daily diet.

Vitamins help the body convert carbohydrates and fat into energy and assist in the formation of bones and tissues. Vitamins are either fat-soluble or water-soluble. Fat-soluble vitamins cannot be dissolved in water, so they are store in the body fat until they are transported to cells by the blood. Because these vitamins can accumulate in the body, it is especially important for a person's regular daily nutrient intake of fat-soluble vitamins not to exceed the tolerable upper intake levels (UL). Water-soluble vitamins must be replenished frequently.

There are eight B vitamins, Thiamin (b-1), riboflavin (B-2), Niacin (B-3), pantothenic acid (B-5), Pyridoxine (B-6), Cobalamin (B-12), Biotin, Folate (folic acid folacin). And the other vitamins are vitamin A, C, D, E, and K. All are necessary for numerous special functions in the body.

THE SMITH'S HIERARCHY OF NUTRITION
©

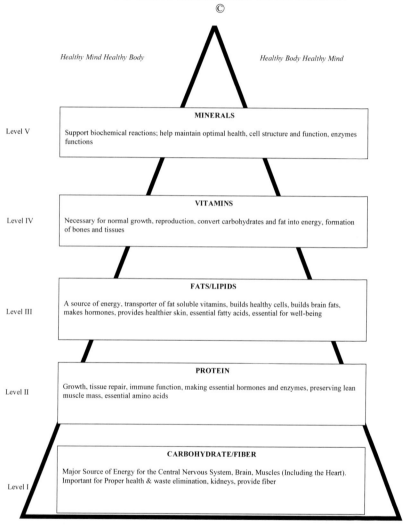

Healthy Mind Healthy Body   *Healthy Body Healthy Mind*

Level V

MINERALS

Support biochemical reactions; help maintain optimal health, cell structure and function, enzymes functions

Level IV

VITAMINS

Necessary for normal growth, reproduction, convert carbohydrates and fat into energy, formation of bones and tissues

Level III

FATS/LIPIDS

A source of energy, transporter of fat soluble vitamins, builds healthy cells, builds brain fats, makes hormones, provides healthier skin, essential fatty acids, essential for well-being

Level II

PROTEIN

Growth, tissue repair, immune function, making essential hormones and enzymes, preserving lean muscle mass, essential amino acids

Level I

CARBOHYDRATE/FIBER

Major Source of Energy for the Central Nervous System, Brain, Muscles (Including the Heart). Important for Proper health & waste elimination, kidneys, provide fiber

Level V: Minerals

Minerals are chemical elements that are vital for life. The body is not equipped to produce the minerals that are needed to function. Instead, these nutrients must be obtained from food. Your health is dependent upon the food choices that you make. Therefore, we must make wise choices. Minerals are as important to the human body as breathing; without the proper amount of minerals, our body would cease to function properly, and if the deficiency is severe enough, it can and will result in death.

Minerals also have a tremendous effect on several of our organs as well as our blood tissue and cells. Maintaining a harmonious balance inside the body is crucial to proper function. If this critical balance of alkaline and acidity gets thrown off, even in the slightest, it can cause chaos in the body known as metabolic imbalance, and this condition can lead to several other life-threatening conditions.

Again, I cannot emphasize enough the necessity for eating the proper foods, and you can never get the proper nutrients, vitamins, and minerals from anything that is not natural, and by that, I mean anything that is not manmade; it is not natural, synthetic. Your food is the way of life.

Look at it this way: a car is more than just looks. You get in it and drive it, but there is so much more to the car. The Maslow chart is the mental, and it relates to how the car you feel in the car, the way it looks, the color, and the way that it drives. The USDA chart is the physical, and it refers to the engine, breaks, alternators, transmission, and components that come together in order for the car to work properly.

The Smith's Hierarchy charts are the biology of life. These charts are related to the gas, oil, transmission fluid, brake fluid, and power steering fluid we need for our cars. They take into account the breath we take and the heartbeat. It is the very essence of life. It is what you can't see; hence sometimes you ignore it and fail to believe it exists. However, if it is not present, there is no life.

The body is like a car: you need fuel in order to function properly. In the case of the car, if you put the wrong gas in the tank, the car will break down, and you will have a lot of operational problems. Also, it will never run correctly as long as you continue to put the wrong type of gas in it. The car will always be in the shop, needing problems fixed, one after another. Your body is just like that poor car! We fuel our body with the foods we eat and beverages we drink. By eating the wrong types of food, we cause our body to stop functioning properly. We continue to eat highly processed, nutrient-lacking foods that lead to sickness and disease, and we pay many visits to the doctor.

Notice the parallel between the Maslow chart with the other charts; they are different, yet they are the same. They are more interrelated rather than sharply separated. The way we eat, what we eat, and how we eat all depends on how we feel about ourselves, our environment, our peers, our upbringing, and our self-respect.

It is essential that we follow the steps of the USDA and the Smith's Hierarchy charts. As you notice, if you follow the Smith's chart, you will see that it is the pure nutrients that your body craves and that are innate for life, that nutrients/nutrition are the force of life.

If you take notice of the nutrient/nutrition charts, you will realize that the only reason that you have been sick, overweight, or underweight is because you have not given your body the proper nutrients/nutrition.

Failure to Thrive

These four hierarchy pyramids, or what I like to call Life Charts, are more interrelated than they are not, and the similarities are great. I will attempt to explain to you where, how, and why these pyramids play a role in everything that we have talked about in this book. These charts represent the beginning and the ending of life and all that is between. Each message is the same, yet they are expressed in a different way; they all deal with the pure essence of life, mental, physical, and biological—all of the intangibles. I will explain to you what correlation I see between these "needs" pyramids. I will show how they are related and just how intricate they are.

There is no life without the basis of what each pyramid represents. Maslow's focuses on the mental, the USDA chart focuses on the physical, and the Smith's focuses on the biological. All are equally important. If you remove either one of these functions of life from the equation, life will cease to exist. Of these charts, the most important thing to note is that the foundation starts with food, as food is your source of nutrients, and nutrition and without nutrients, nothing is able to exist.

These pyramids are put together to explain the necessity of how important each component is. With each pyramid, you begin at the bottom or the base at level one and work your way up. Maslow says we must attempt to try to complete each step in order to thrive; otherwise, we will fail to thrive. We are always in a delayed stage. This is called Failure to Thrive. Therefore, we must continue in levels, understanding that each level is important and need each other to be complete. It is like you need all body parts. You need the neck in order to support the head, and you need your chest top support the neck, etc. I consider level one to be like a sleeping volcano because it is often overlooked or ignored. We do not realize what is brewing beneath until it erupts. At this point, it has zapped the life from us because we can't see and don't even know that they exist. Level one is very important, as it is the basis for all things that make us.

Each pyramid shows how moving from one level to the next level in life, whether it is mental, physical, or biological, can affect your function in another realm of life. For example, in the nutrients chart, if you fail to get the enzymes your body needs, then even eating all the "right" foods will have no benefit because you failed to have ingested what it takes to make them work. If you do not obtain enzymes in your diet, then you are not thriving biologically. The proper balance of the "right" foods—food high in nutrients—is so vital to life. Without this balance, we are in a state of "Failure to Thrive." We are a society of nations filled with people with Failure to Thrive.

Failure to Thrive has long been associated with infants who do not gain weight or grow in height according to their peers. The elderly can develop a syndrome called acute brain syndrome. This syndrome shows symptoms of a gradual decline in physical and/or mental functioning along with weight loss, decreased appetite, and withdrawal from social interactions in the absence of an explanation for these symptoms.

Failure to Thrive occurs at the beginning of life, while acute brain syndrome occurs toward the end of life. Nonetheless, it is my belief that they both occur because of malnutrition. You simply cannot move from a level until you have satisfied the level you are in, and this is where the Failure to Thrive comes into play. Infants cannot thrive if his or her very basic needs are not met; this leads to impaired cognitive skills, independence, etc.

In the elderly, the individual begins to decline because of years of the wrong foods, and they begin to deteriorate. They have loss of muscle skills, and they depend on others for their very basic needs. It is a cycle. The end of life does not have to be like the beginning if individuals would take charge of their own body and simply eat foods with nutrition and nutrients, as this changes everything about life.

Problems including physical, social, mental, and environmental difficulties, along with severely diminished coping abilities and functional capacities, all go back to proper nutrition and nutrients. What does this have to do with weight and nutrition? Everything. Without certain nutrients, there is no life beginning with the mitochondria in our cells. Our body is made of trillions of living cells, and without living food, the cells die; therefore, we die.

Weight management and good health is vital (essential) to life. The loss of weight should be about good health. To look good is to feel good. Therefore, when you lose weight, you want it to be done in a healthy manner. Weight loss in an unhealthy manner can result in you looking old with sagging skin, joint pain, and stomach problems. If you look older and have no energy, you have just defeated your purpose for losing weight. For this reason, if you want to have great weight, look great, and feel great, then you must do it the *healthy* way. When losing weight, you want to improve your quality of life with longevity not to decrease it. To look good is to feel good.

One of the first things that happen as people age is there is a decline in muscle mass, muscle strength, and endurance. Associated with this muscle decline, there is a decline in aerobic capacity, resulting in people become easily fatigued. This decline begins in the thirties with rapid deterioration in the mid-sixties. This is why it is so important to get the proper nutrients as soon as possible. However, it is never too late to start, as later is better than not at all. Eating the proper nutrients can slow down and even begin to reverse the aging process. Your aging process, health, and quality of life are all about the food you eat.

Muscle protein production begins to naturally slow down in people when they age. Muscle proteins are the functional molecules that have specific tasks. The decrease in muscle protein production can impact on muscle functions. The age at which it begins and the rate at which it progresses depends on an individual's genetic makeup and level of physical activity. Muscle fibers also decline with age. Fewer muscle fibers translate into reduced numbers of components from which to make muscles. The result: less muscles mass. As muscle and its protein content diminish, they become fatigued more easily.

Dr. Nair's research shows that sarcopenia is intimately involved in activating the aging process. In particular, a reaction within tiny intracellular organelles called mitochondria appears to be a powerful determinant of sarcopenia and other physical changes the body experiences as it ages. Mayo Clinic Endocrinologist K. Seekuman Nair, PhD, MD is a leading researcher on muscle metabolism and its role in aging. He also is director of Mayo's CTSA Clinic Research unit (CRU), which is the oldest center of its kind in the country and is funded by the National Institutes of Health (NIH).

An organism takes in nutrients from the food it digests. Food is converted into chemical energy in the form of ATP (a complex chemical process called oxidative phosphorylation) in every tissue. ATP is the currency of a cell and is the key energy form needed for all cellular functions. This process of ATP formation takes place in tiny organelles within each cell known as mitochondria, which are the powerhouses of the cell. For muscles to perform its mechanical functions, ATP must be converted to ADP to release chemical energy into mechanical energy. ATP is also essential for remodeling tissues and other various life maintaining functions. In fact, a shortage of ATP results in eventual dysfunction of organs.

Dr. Nair explains that once you lose muscle mass, metabolic syndrome begins. Muscle is one of the major organs involved in metabolism and in setting the body's metabolic rate and fuel burning following a meal. When a person loses activity and loses muscle mass, and if they continue to maintain caloric intake, they become overweight, especially in the abdominal region. This excess weight contributes to glucose intolerance or resistance to insulin action.

I am convinced that there are only two ways to gain weight, become sick, or even age, and they are the *outer* and the *inner*.

The *outer* consists of items outside our body like the food we eat, what we drink (including water), and the substances we breathe. The *inner* is how these *outer* items are processed and/or absorbed in our bodies as well as what remains undigested.

Take a look at your daily routine. Are you inhaling harmful chemical substances like household cleaning products or cigarette smoke? Are your foods full of unnatural preservatives? Something as simple as this can cause free radicals within your body. These free radicals can damage your cells and ATP production. Now you have caused yourself to prematurely age!

Food is the way people attempt to control what they are feeling. Food has become a way to try to fill a void in life and a way to make up for what they may or may not feel. All the while not realizing that they are eating empty calories and food with no nutrients. Eating these wrong types of food can lead to more health problems. These foods suppress the immune system and hormones that trigger the brain. This can alter your mental state of well being, and you continue to eat wrong food. This leads to mental incapacity.

All mental disorders, eating disorders, depression, bipolarism, and physical disorders all come from the same root. I call it food disorder. You eat because you are depressed, and you are depressed because you are eating; it's just a repeated cycle. Mental problems are eating problems. All people are in one phase or the other; either you eat or you do not eat because of a mental problem, whether it is emotional, depression, lonely, self-esteem issues, worthiness issues, etc.

What you eat or do not eat has a great effect on your mental state; missing the proper nutrients affect your whole being physically, biologically, spiritually, mentally, and emotionally. Food is *life*. The wrong food is death.

CONCLUSION

American society has recently experienced a prolonged era of progressive obesity in our population with associated worsening of the general health of the population. There is a nationwide rampant increase in the medical conditions associated with diet. These conditions are diabetes, hypertension, metabolic syndromes, steatohepatitis due to fatty liver, arteriosclerosis with associated stroke, and loss of limbs due to peripheral vascular disease.

One of the most puzzling facts of modern times is that while American Society has continued to prosper and our basic standard of living has improved on all levels, the general health of the population has deteriorated. We can make great strides in improving our overall well being if we would just focus on proper nutrition. Instead we expend valuable time, effort and finances on dieting and pay very little attention to wellness and preventive health. If the billions of dollars spent on dieting was spent on buying and preparing the proper food, our society would be much healthier.

So in summary Americans have become obsessed with fad diets, starving themselves, overeating, and under eating. America has become a society of the mal-nourished. Even those that are eating are eating foods with no nutrition because they are so caught up with counting calories, while ignoring the value of nutrients.

According to the USDA an adequate and balanced diet should provide all necessary nutrients, without the need for dieting supplements. Real, natural, and organic food trumps anything that is processed, chemi-cally changed or synthetic. Dr. Howell states that it is impossible to gain weight from raw fruits and vegetable no matter how much you eat, because the body will absorb it in a different way for use and not store it as fat (Howell).

People should stop counting calories and begin to focus more on nutrients and nutrition and how the body absorbs them.

APPENDIX

Amino acid: the building block for proteins containing a central carbon atom with nitrogen and other atoms attached.

Antioxidants: substances or nutrients in our foods that can prevent or slow the oxidative damage to our body. When our body cells use oxygen, they naturally produce free radicals (by product), which can cause damage. Antioxidants act as free radicals.

Balanced diet: simply means that you provide your body with all of the basic nutrients that it needs to provide you with energy each day as well as to repair and build tissue.

Carbohydrates: the body's primary sources for fuel, with the exception of some isolated populations (such as those who traditionally subsisted primarily on fats and proteins), carbohydrates comprise the majority of calories in most modern human diets.

Simple Carbohydrates: includes sugars like sucrose (table sugar), fructose (fruit sugar), and grape sugars, which are glucose or dextrose. Of the three types of simple sugars, glucose and dextrose are the most easily digested and used for energy.

Complex Carbohydrates: contain three or more linked sugars and thus require the body to work harder to break them down into glucose for energy. Some complex carbohydrates, like fruit or vegetable fibers, for example, cannot be broken down by the body and are passed through undigested.

Carotenoids: pigment materials in fruits and vegetables that orange color from yellow to orange to red, three of the various carotenoids yield vitamin A. Many are antioxidants.

Energy: the capacity of body or physical system for doing work.

Energy Balance: a measurement of the biological homeostasis of energy in living systems. It is the state in which the total energy intake equals total energy needs. It is the difference between calorie intake (from food and drinks) and calories out through our metabolism and energy expended during daily activities.

Positive Energy Balance: a condition in which more energy is taken in as food than is expended during metabolism; body weight increases and fat stores are increased as a result.

Negative Energy Balance: a situation in which a person is using more energy on a day-to-day basis than he/she consumes, leading to weight loss.

Enzyme: a compound that speeds the rate of a chemical reaction but is not altered by the reaction; almost all enzymes are protein (some are made of genetic material).

Fatty acid: major part of most lipids, primarily composed of a chain of carbons flanked by hydrogen.

Saturated fatty acid: a fatty acid containing no carbon-carbon double bonds.

Unsaturated fatty acid: a fatty acid containing one or more carbon-carbon double bonds.

Fructose: natural sugar present in onions, artichokes, pears, and wheat.

Glucose: a six-carbon monosaccharide that usually exists in a ring form, found as such in blood and in table sugar bonded to fructose, also known as dextrose. It is the sugar that the body makes from the three elements of food—proteins, fats, and carbohydrates—but mostly from carbohydrates. Glucose is the major source of energy for living cells.

High fructose corn syrup (HFCS): manufactured using genetically modified organisms, it is not natural. It is manufactured through a chemical process that breaks down natural components of sugars, extracts and converts the remaining compounds in to industrially usable substances, and then recombines the usable bits to make a viscous syrup. It is par for the course for industrial food breakdown of natural foods into individual components, strip out what they consider usable in the manufacturing process, fundamentally change it with more chemical processing, and then recombine it into something that sells. It is manmade and synthetic. There is nothing natural about it (almostfit.com). Dr. Robert Lustig calls it "white poison."

Insoluble Fiber: form of fiber that passes essentially unchanged through the intestines and produces little gas; wheat bran and some vegetables contain this kind of fiber.

Lactose: natural sugar in milk; it is also found in milk products, such as cheese and ice cream and processed foods; bread; cereal; and salad dressing.

Macronutrient: a nutrient needed in large quantities in a diet (protein, fats, and carbohydrates).

Maltose (or malt sugar): a disaccharide formed from two units of glucose joined with an a (1-4) bond. Maltose is the disaccharide produced when amylase breaks down starch. It is found in germinating seeds, such as barley, as they break down their starch to use for food. It is also produced when glucose is caramelized.

Melatonin: a natural hormone in all living creatures, from plants to animals. In higher animal species, it is produced in the pineal gland (in the brain) but also in the eye (retina) and the gastro-intestinal tract. Melatonin also plays a key role in memory and our ability to learn quickly.

Metabolic: of or relating to metabolism, "metabolic rate."

Metabolism: the set of chemical reactions that happen in living organisms to maintain life. These processes allow organisms to grow and reproduce, maintain their structures, and respond to their environments.

Micronutrient: a nutrient needed in small quantities in a diet (vitamins and minerals).

Mineral: element used in the body to promote chemical reactions and to form body structures.

Mitochondria: Normal structures responsible for energy production in cells; called the powerhouse of the cell because their primary purpose is to manufacture adenosine triphosphate (ATP), which is used as a source of energy.

Mucosa: the membranes (or mucosea, singular mucosa) are linings of mostly endodermal origin, covered in epithelium, which are involved in absorption and secretion. They line various body cavities that are exposed to the external environment and internal organs.

Organelle: refers to different bodies within a living cell that perform various functions (e.g. vacuole, endoplasmic reticulum). Organelles are a specialized subunit within a cell that has a specific function and is usually separately enclosed within its own lipid bilayer.

Phytochemical: a chemical found in plants some phytochemicals may contribute to a reduced risk of cancer or cardiovascular disease in people who consume them regularly.

Protein: a food and body components made of amino acids, protein contain carbon, hydrogen, little oxygen, nitrogen, and sometimes other atoms, in a specific configuration.

Complete Proteins: contain all nine essential amino acids that the body cannot otherwise produce on its own. With the exception of soybeans, complete proteins are only found in animal foods like meat, poultry, fish, eggs, and milk and dairy products.

Incomplete Proteins: lack one or more the nine essential amino acids. Incomplete sources of protein include most vegetables, as well as nuts, beans, seed, peas, and grains. Soybeans, however, are a complete protein.

Raffinose: complex sugar found largely in beans; smaller amounts are amounts in cabbage, Brussels sprouts, broccoli asparagus, other vegetables, and whole grains.

Sarcopenia (from the Greek meaning "poverty of flesh"): the degenerative loss of skeletal muscle mass and strength associated with aging. Sarcopenia is a component of the frailty syndrome.

Serotonin: a hormone manufactured by the brain, serotonin is a feel-good chemical that, along with dopamine, has been shown to have antioxidant properties. Serotonin is involved in mood and behavior, physical coordination, appetite, body temperature, and sleep.

Sorbitol: a form of sugar naturally found in fruits, including apples, pears and peaches, and prunes; it is also used as an artificial sweetener in many dietetic foods and sugar-free candies and gums.

Soluble Fiber: fiber that dissolves easily in water and takes on a soft, gel-like texture in the intestines; (found in oat bran, beans, peas, and most fruits) it is not broken down.

Starches: produce gas as they are broken down in the large intestine; they include potatoes, corn, pasta, and wheat. Rice is the only starch that does not cause gas.

Sucrose: table sugar. It is equally destructive as fructose, which can only be metabolized by the liver chronically raised insulin. Fructose and sucrose have the same effect on the body (cause fatty liver etc.).

Triglyceride: the major form of lipid in the body and in food. It is composed of three fatty acids bonded to glycerol.

Trace mineral: a mineral vital to health that is required in the diet in amounts less than 100 milligrams per day.

Trans fat: formed by the hydrogenation of vegetable oils and has been shown to raise cholesterol and heart disease risk.

Unsaturated Fat: a fatty acid containing one or more carbon-carbon double bonds.

A fat that is liquid at room temperature and comes from a plant such as olive, peanut, corn, cottonseed, sunflower, safflower, or soybean. Unsaturated fats tend to lower the level of cholesterol in the blood.

Monounsaturated Fat: a fatty acid containing one carbon-carbon double bond.

Polyunsaturated Fat: a fatty acid containing two or more carbon-carbon double bond.

Vitamin: a compound needed in very small amounts in the diet to help regulate and support chemical reactions in the body.

Fat-soluble vitamins: dissolve in fat and such substances as either and benzene but not readily in water. These vitamins are A, D, E and K.

Water-soluble vitamins: dissolve in water, these vitamins are the B vitamins and vitamin C.

Whole grains: contains the entire seed of the plant, including the bran, germ, and endosperm (starchy interior). Examples are whole wheat and brown rice.

ABOUT THE AUTHOR

Mrs. Louise Moore Smith is the founder and CEO of Smith's Nutrition Products, INC. She has over thirty years of experience in medical service and medical service administration. She served her country as a communication specialist in the United States Army. As she advanced, she served as a medic/EMT and nurse. She has worked for Boeing Aircraft Company as a flight and computer testing administrator for 757 and 767 aircrafts. Louise holds Bachelor of Science degrees in Early Elementary Education, and Child Development from North Carolina Agricultural and Technical State University. She furthered her studies in Theology and Church Ministry from John Wesley and Winston Salem Bible Colleges. Mrs. Smith, along with her husband Dr. LeRoy Smith, co-founded Rockingham Medical and Surgical Associates, where she has served as chief executive officer and office administrator.

She has extensive research in Holistic Health and is an avid practicing believer of holistic and spiritual healing. Over the past four years, she has done intensive and extensive literature research on non-traditional therapeutic practices.

She has been married to Dr. LeRoy C. Smith, MD for twenty-nine years and is the proud mother of two amazing children: daughter, Nathaina and son, LeRoy II.

BIBLIOGRAPHY

Lustig, MD, Robert. "Sugar: The Bitter Truth." Recorded July 27, 2009. UC San Francisco. Web, http://www.uctv.tv/search-details.aspx?showID=16717.

Howell, Edward. *Food Enzymes for Health and Longetivity 2nd Edition*. Twin Lakes, WI: Lotus Press, 1994.

Chichoke, Anthony. *Enzymes & Enzyme Therapy: How to Jump-start Your Way to lifelong good health*. Chicago, IL: Keats Publishing, 2000.

Kirschmann, John. *Nutrition Almanac 6th Edition*. New York, NY: McGraw-Hill, 2007.

Wardlaw, Gordon, and Anne Smith. *Contemporary Nutrition 7th Edition*. New York, NY: McGraw- Hill, 2006.

Clapp, Larry. *Prostate Health in 90 Days*. Maui, Hawaii: Hay House, 1997.

Campbell, Colin, and Thomas Campbell II. The China Study: Startling Implictions for Diet, Weight Loss, and Long-term Health. Dallas, TX: Benbella Books, INC, 2006.

Mateljon, George. The World's Healthiest Foods: Essential Guide for the healthiest way of eating. Seattle, WA: George Mateljon Foundation, 2007.

Schauss, Alexander. *Mineral, Trace Elements, and Human Health 4th Edition*. Tacoma, WA: Biosocial Publications, 1995.

Shils, Maurice, James Olson, and Moshe Shike. *Modern Nutrition in Health and Disease Vol2. 8th Edition*. Malvern, PA: Lea & Febiger, 1994.

Bender, David. *Nutritional Biochemistry of the Vitamins*. New York, NY: Cambridge University Press, 2003.

Parker, Steve. *The Human Body Book*. New York, NY: DK Publishing, 2007.

Maslow, Abraham. "A Theory of Human Motivation." *Psychological Review*. 50. no. 4 (1943): 370-396.

PubMED Health: A.D. a.m. Medical Encyclopedia, "Failure to thrive." http://www.ncbi.nlm.nih.gov/pubmedhealth/PMH0001986/.

PubMED Health: A.D. a.m. Medical Encyclopedia, "Acute Brain Syndrome." http://www.ncbi.nlm.nih.gov/pubmedhealth/PMH0001749/

US Department of Health and Human Services, "Quick Guide to Healthy Living: Nutrition and Fitness." http://www.healthfinder.gov/prevention/category.aspx?catId=1.

HealthyPeople.gov. US Department of Health and Human Services , "Nutrition and Weight Status." http://www.healthypeople.gov/2020/topicsobjectives2020/overview.aspx?topicid=29.

Office of Disease Prevention and Health Promtion, First. US Department of Health and Human Services, "Office of Disease Prevention and Health Promotion, U.S. Department of Health and Human Services–ODPHP." http://www.healthfinder.gov/orgs/HR2013.htm.

Office of Dietary Supplements: National Institute of Health, "Dietary Supplement Fact Sheet: Folate." Last modified April 15, 2009. Accessed November 13, 2010. http://ods.od.nih.gov/factsheets/folate/.

Office of Dietary Supplements: National Institute of Health, "Dietary Supplement Fact Sheet: Vitamin D." http://ods.od.nih.gov/factsheets/vitamind/

Office of Dietary Supplements: National Institute of Health, "Dietary Supplement Fact Sheet: Vitamin D:Quick-facts." http://ods.od.nih.gov/factsheets/VitaminD-QuickFacts/.

United States Department of Agriculture, "Tips for Eating Healthy When Eating Out." Last modified May 27, 2011. http://www.choosemyplate.gov/tipsresources/eating_out.html

United States Department of Agriculture, "USDA's Food Guide Pyramid Booklet 1992." Accessed September 8, 2010. http://www.cnpp.usda.gov/Publications/MyPyramid/OriginalFoodGuidePyramids/FGP/FGPPamphlet.pdf.

USDA: Agriculture Research Service, "Food and Nutrition Research Briefs Jan 2005." Last modified February 14, 2007. Accessed October 18, 2010. http://www.ars.usda.gov/is/np/fnrb/fnrb0105.htm.

US Food and Drug Administration, "Make your Calories Count." Last modified March 11, 2011. Accessed October 09, 2010. http://www.fda.gov/Food/LabelingNutrition/ConsumerInformation/ucm114022.htm.

Center for Disease Control and Prevention, "Fruit and Vegetable Benefits." Accessed October 09, 2010. http://fruitsandveggiesmatter.gov/benefits/index.HMTL .

Center for Disease Control and Prevention, "Nutrition for Everyone: Basics: Carbohydrates." Accessed November 13, 2010. http://www.cdc.gov/nutrition/everyone/basics/carbs.html.

Christen, WG, JM Gaziano, and CH Hennekens. "Design of Physicians' Health Study II—a randomized trial of beta-carotene, vitamins E and C, and multivitamins, in prevention of cancer, cardiovascular disease, and eye disease, and review of results of completed trials." *Annals of Epidemology.* 10. no. 2 (2000): 125-34.

Song, Y, NR Cook, CM Albert, M Van Denburgh, and JE Manson. "Effects of vitamins C and E and beta-carotene on the risk of type 2 diabetes in women at high risk of cardiovascular disease: a randomized controlled trial.." *American Journal of Clinical Nutrition.* 90. no. 2 (2009): 429-37. http://www.ncbi.nlm.nih.gov/pubmed?term=19491386 (accessed November 6, 2010).

Manson, JE, JM Gaziano, A Spelsberg, p.m.Ridker, NR Cook, JE Buring, and WC Willett. "A secondary prevention trial of antioxidant vitamins and cardiovascular disease in women. Rationale, design, and methods. The WACS Research Group." *Annals of Epidemology.* 5. no. 4 (1995): 261-9. http://www.ncbi.nlm.nih.gov/pubmed?term=8520707 (accessed November 7, 2010).

Cook, NR, CM Albert, JM Gaziano, E Zaharris, J MacFadyen, E Danielson, JE Buring and JE Manson. "A randomized factorial trial of vitamins C and E and beta carotene in the secondary prevention of cardiovascular events in women: results from the Women's Antioxidant Cardiovascular Study." *Archives of Internal Medicine*. 168. no. 7 (2008): 1610-18.

Shapiro, Alexandra, Wei Mu, Carlos Roncal, Kit-Yan Cheng, Richard Johnson, and Philip Scarpace. "Fructose-induced leptin resistance exacerbates weight gain in response to subsequent high-fat feeding ." *American Journal of Physiology*. 295. no. 5 (2008): R1370-75.

National Institutes of Health State-of-the-Science Panel. "NIH State-of-the-Science Conference Statement on Multivitamin/Mineral Supplements and Chronic Disease Prevention." *American Journal of Clinical Nutrition*. 85. no. 1 (2007): 257S-64S.

Enig, Mary G. 1993. "Fats & Oils: Understanding the Functions and Properties of Partially Hydrogenated Fats and Oils and Their Relationship to Unhydrogenated Fats and Oils." *Townsend Letter for Doctors & Patients* no. 125: 1212.

Norris, Jeffery. University of San Francisco, "Sugar is a Poison, says UCSF Obesity Expert." Last modified June 25, 2009. Accessed November 12, 2011. http://www.ucsf.edu/science-cafe/articles/obesity-and-metabolic-syndrome-driven-by-fructose-sugar-diet/.

Group, Edward. Global Healing Center, "5 Health Dangers of High Fructose Corn Syrup." Last modified July 8, 2010. Accessed October 12, 2011. http://www.globalhealingcenter.com/natural-health/high-fructose-corn-syrup-dangers/.

Fife, Bruce. "Things You Probably Didn't Know About Coconut Oil." *Healthy Living Magazine*. http://www.coconutresearchcenter.org/article10013.htm.

Jordan, Jo. Puristat: Digestive Wellness Center, "What is the function of the Colon?." Puristat.com/colon-cleansing/colonfunction.aspx.

Puristat: Digestive Wellness Center, "Can a liver cleanse help your liver function more efficiently?." Accessed March 13, 2010. http://www.puristat.com/liver-cleansing/default.aspx.

Hepatitis B Foundation, "Your Liver and its Functions." Last modified October 21, 2009. Accessed January 20, 2009. http://www.hepb.org/hepb/your_liver.htm.

Diet.com: Your Nutrition and Health Solution, "Negative Calorie Diet." Accessed October 12, 2011. http://www.diet.com/g/negative-calorie-diet.

Decuypere, J.D. "Dr. Decuypere's Nutrient Charts." Accessed March 9, 2009. http://healthalternatives2000.com/vitamins-nutrition-chart.html.

The Cancer Cure Foundation, "Cancer Fighting Foods/Spices ." http://www.cancure.org/cancer_fighting_foods.htm.

Preventive-Health-Guide.com, "You need the right balance of vitamins and minerals.." Last modified 2008. Accessed November 2, 2010. http://www.preventive-health-guide.com/vitamins-and-minerals.html.

IrishHealth.com, "The Role of Vitamins and Minerals." Accessed March 9, 2009. http://www.irishhealth.com/clin/ffl/vitamin.html.

IrishHealth.com, "Probiotics and your health." Accessed March 10, 2009. http://www.irishhealth.com/clin/ffl/probiotics.html

ScienceDaily, "When it comes to Red Cabbage, more is better." Last modified March 11, 2008. Accessed February 20, 2009. http://www.sciencedaily.com/releases/2008/03/080307081409.

ACRIA, "Keeping You Liver Healthy." http://www.the-body.com/content/art14306.html.

Leonard, Vaughnlea. "How does the body control Blood Sugar Levels." Accessed October 29, 2009. http://www.ehow.com/how-does_5004461_body-control-blood-sugar-levels.html.

Wilcox, Christie. Nutrition Wonderland, "Understanding Our Bodies: Leptin (The Fullness Hormone)." Last modified June 15, 2009. Accessed January 30, 2011. http://nutritionwonderland.com/2009/06/understanding-our-bodies-leptin-the-fullness-hormone/.

International Hyperhidrosis, "Hyperhidrosis Treatments: Botox Injections." Accessed December 12, 2010. http://www.sweathelp.org/English/PFF_Treatment_Injections.asp.